The Journey Within Embracing Perimenopause

By

Lucy Connor

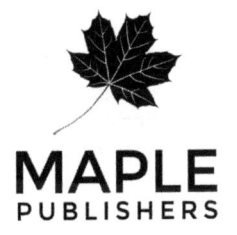

MAPLE
PUBLISHERS

The Journey Within: Navigating Perimenopause

Author: Lucy Connor

Copyright © 2024 Lucy Connor

The right of Lucy Connor to be identified as author of this work has been asserted by the author in accordance with section 77 and 78 of the Copyright, Designs and Patents Act 1988.

First Published in 2024

ISBN 978-1-83538-411-4 (Paperback)
978-1-83538-412-1 (Hardback)
978-1-83538-413-8 (E-Book)

Book Cover Design and Book Layout by:
White Magic Studios
www.whitemagicstudios.co.uk

Published by:
Maple Publishers
Fairbourne Drive, Atterbury,
Milton Keynes,
MK10 9RG, UK
www.maplepublishers.com

A CIP catalogue record for this title is available from the British Library.

All rights reserved. No part of this book may be reproduced or translated in any form or by any means, electronic or mechanical, including photocopying, recording or by any information storage and retrieval system without written permission from the author.

The views expressed in this work are solely those of the author and do not necessarily reflect the publisher's opinions, and the publisher, as a result of this, disclaims any responsibility for them.

CONTENTS

Dedication 5

Acknowledgments 6

Introduction 8

Chapter 1 – Understanding the Change 12
    What Exactly is Perimenopause? 17
    When Does Perimenopause Occur? 18
    Signs and Symptoms of Perimenopause 18
    The Role of Hormones During Perimenopause 22

Chapter 2 – Navigating the Physical Changes 25
    Hormonal Fluctuations 26
    Menstrual Changes 29
    Hot Flashes and Night Sweats 32
    Weight Gain and Metabolism Changes 34
    Bone Health 36
    Skin and Hair Changes 37
    Breast Health 40

Chapter 3 – The Emotional Rollercoaster During Perimenopause 42
    Hormonal Impact on Emotions 42
    Mood Swings and Irritability 46
    Anxiety and Depression 49
    Brain Fog 51
    Self-Care and Stress Management 54
    Communication and Support 60

Chapter 4 – Nurturing Relationships During Perimenopause 64
    Your Relationship With Yourself 64
    Communication with Loved Ones............................... 66
    Explaining Changes in Libido and Intimacy 68

Chapter 5 – Lifestyle Changes for Optimal Wellbeing 71
    Nutrition and Diet.. 72
    Regular Exercise 77
    Sleep Hygiene 82
    Stress Management... 87
    Mindfulness and Relaxation 92

Chapter 6 – Seeking Support and Professional Guidance.. 96
    Healthcare Professional Guidance.............................. 98
    Mental Health Support 106
    Support Groups and Online Communities 109

Chapter 7 – Hormonal and Non-Hormonal Treatment Options 113
    Understanding HRT 114
    Alternative Therapies 122

Chapter 8 – Conclusion...132

Chapter 9 – References...135

Chapter 10 – Appendices..137
    Appendix 1: Perimenopause Symptom Tracker.137
    Appendix 2: Questions for Your Healthcare Provider...139
    Appendix 3: Medication Tracker 140
    Appendix 4: Relaxation Techniques.........................142

Dedication

To all the remarkable women walking the winding path of perimenopause, this book is for you. May you find strength in every step, and comfort in knowing that you are not alone on this journey.

To the spouses and partners who stand beside them, this is your guide—a source of understanding and a reminder of the love that binds you. May it light the way as you support your beloved through this profound transformation.

We walk this path together, hand in hand, heart to heart.

Acknowledgments

First and foremost, I extend my deepest gratitude to the most high God, for granting me the opportunity and the courage to bring this long-held dream to life. It is by His grace that I've been able to believe in myself and finally set pen to paper, turning a distant dream into reality.

To my beloved husband, words cannot fully express my appreciation for your unwavering support throughout this journey. Thank you for standing by me with patience and understanding as I navigate the countless changes during this transitional phase of my life. Your encouragement has been my anchor, and I am endlessly grateful.

To my wonderful sons, Tyrese and Jordan, I am blessed beyond measure to be your mother. Your love, understanding, and support have been a source of strength for me as I ventured through this unfamiliar terrain. Your kindness and care remind me daily how fortunate I am, and I am so proud to be your mum.

To my Jamaican mother, Veronica Wynter, you are a blessing beyond words. You have been a beacon of love and strength for me and my family, embodying the same caring nature as my late Mum. Sometimes, I truly believe she handpicked you from heaven to guide me when she became an angel herself. You have stood by me through it all, offering your unwavering support, your wise counsel, and your warm embrace during my weakest moments. I am forever grateful for your love, your herbs that have soothed my symptoms, and your constant reassurance that I can navigate this journey with grace. Looking at you in your sixties—so vibrant, full of life, and healthy—fills me with hope and admiration. Thank you, Mum, from the depths of my heart.

To my cherished female friends, both younger and of my age, let us arm ourselves with the knowledge and understanding of perimenopause. Together, we can thrive through it, viewing it not as a hindrance but as a step towards greater well-being.

To my dear childhood friend, Ann Kisese, thank you for sharing your journey with me, for your openness, and for your unwavering support. Our conversations have been a lifeline, a space where we compare notes, check in on each other, and offer mutual understanding. Your willingness to listen without judgment has been a gift, and I am truly grateful for your friendship.

Introduction

Perimenopause hits you hard. First come the hot flashes. Then insomnia. Then depression. As you struggle to express the changes happening to you, you come up against a culture of silence. All through history, the natural physical transition of perimenopause (and menopause) has been thought of as something to deny, eradicate and fear. This is strange because women constitute about 51% of the global population. Virtually all of them will experience perimenopause and menopause when that time comes, and still the hormonal changes they experience are taboo to talk about?

According to research done by Bonafide in 2021 (a company that sells products to address women's health conditions), relatively few women talk about their perimenopause symptoms. They conducted a study with 1039 women aged between 40 and 65 in the United States and found that 29% of them never looked for information about perimenopause before they experienced it. 45% of them didn't know the difference between perimenopause – the transition leading to menopause – and menopause itself, the biological process marking the end of a woman's menstrual cycle.

Of the women who were surveyed, 20% had experienced symptoms for more than a year before getting assessed by a healthcare provider and 34% had never formally sought help. Surprisingly, 73% of them did not know how to treat their symptoms including weight gain, hot flashes, sleep difficulties and night sleep. In my personal experience, it has been that if anyone has any expectations or knowledge of what the perimenopause transition will be like, the most common symptoms are night sweats, hot flashes, mood swings, irritability and brain fog. There is often little preparation for anything else, but it happens. Perimenopause can be scary for some women and liberating for others.

It is expected that by 2025, the number of perimenopausal women worldwide will reach 1.1 billion. How do we ensure that our needs are met? How do we prepare for this inevitable transition? As a woman who is going through perimenopause, and who has watched the effects of silence, I have come to believe that talking about it will make it less daunting and isolating and stigmatizing for all women. That is why I wrote this book.

One day in my mid-40s, I woke up feeling low, and then it kept happening. I didn't let it stop me from doing my life as usual. I kept working, and loving the people in my life.

Then suddenly, I started feeling itchy in my arms and legs. It was the weirdest sensation. I noticed that there was no way to stop the itching – once it started, I would itch for what felt like eternity. The sensation was so intense that I could barely concentrate on anything else. I decided to take an antihistamine to try and control it and to my pleasurable surprise, the itchiness stopped. It was starting to look like a lot of things were wrong with my body – well, except my skin. For some reason, my skin was flawless and glowy. I loved it.

Later that day, I went to pick up my son from school. As I waited for him to come out, I felt my body begin to warm up from my feet. The heat went up all the way to the rest of my body. As it got close to my face, it burst into a sweat. I imagine I looked like I had been running a marathon, which is strange, given I had just arrived in my car. I was taken aback. As I was trying to understand what had just happened, one of my son's teachers who I believe was roughly the same age as me stopped to say hello to me. I will never forget her words to me once she saw the situation 'welcome to my world, Lucy.'

It turned out I had just been introduced to a new world. From there on, I experienced a series of changes that left me completely confused. I tried to find answers to help me navigate but unfortunately, no one seemed to have them. In fact, the subject seemed to make many people uneasy. Even my own elder sisters were unwilling to have the conversation. Meanwhile, I still continued to experience occasional itchiness that would only bow to antihistamines. The hot flashes and night sweats became a common thing and my periods became very heavy. My sexual drive stayed unchanged, but for the first time in my life I experienced vaginal dryness which meant making love was not as enjoyable for me.

After slogging through life for a while, I decided to learn. I took it upon myself to understand what was happening to me and how best I could manage the change. I have always been a reader, having a very curious mind. So, I started reading whatever I could find on menopause and perimenopause. I soon found that there was so much information available if you have the patience to wade through it. I was also struck by how misunderstood a lot of women going through perimenopause are.

One of the shocking realizations was that women between 45 and 55 are easily prescribed antidepressants and sometimes put into mental institutions because of the symptoms they present with. Some of them closely resemble mental disorders. Imagine that. Imagine how confusing, alienating and stigmatizing it must be to experience so much change within yourself, consult a professional and have yourself locked up, only to find out later on that simple lifestyle changes could have helped you manage your symptoms.

In my case, slowly, but surely, I started learning how to manage my symptoms. I was keen to find out how I could eliminate vaginal dryness, for example. Every woman wants to still be able to enjoy intimacy despite her age. In my research, I stumbled upon some natural herbs which I take on a regular basis. Miraculously, they completely eliminated vaginal dryness. I have found it to be the case with many other symptoms of perimenopause – there are ways to deal and manage the changes within so that you don't only survive through perimenopause, but thrive.

This is the reason I wrote this book. I want to shed light on this often misunderstood and under-discussed phase of a woman's life. My goal is to empower you with the knowledge and tools you need to understand and embrace the changes that come with perimenopause. Here, you will find expert advice and practical tips from my research as well as personal stories to help you begin understanding what is happening to you. If I manage to make your transition a little less daunting and a lot more manageable, I will have achieved my goal. If that's what you're looking for, keep reading.

Chapter 1
Understanding the Change

Before we can jump into the biological and practical changes that happen during perimenopause, let me tell you the stories of four women. Read through them and see if there are things that you can relate to and that resonate with your experience. Bear in mind that because each woman's experience is different, no one woman's story will directly be like yours. What we can do is find the parallels, and learn from each other to make our experience less burdensome and more enjoyable.

Jane's Story

Jane's mother, like most of our mothers, taught her about getting her periods but didn't touch on the important stages of perimenopause and menopause. She remembers her grandmother calling it 'the change' but she was only 20 at the time and had no idea what the referred change was. Not so long ago, Jane, a vice principal at a school in London, was enjoying the buzz of the classroom and the pressure of management. She was 40 years old. She was working as a teacher full-time. She had experience teaching and loved every minute of her job.

All of that changed in two years. By the time Jane turned 42, the symptoms of perimenopause forced her to step back from her role at work. She woke up one day and suddenly thought; 'I can't do this.' In the days that followed, she completely lost her confidence. Where she would have stuck up for herself, she felt stuck. She could not shake the negative thoughts about her abilities. The pressure was within and she somehow couldn't get any perspective. Rather than walk around with confidence, she started feeling fearful, until she resigned from her role as deputy. Jane, is like many women, who, after spending many years working in high pressure jobs, end up signing off because of the symptoms of perimenopause.

Ann's Story

Ann started having night sweats at age 34. She did not dive into educating herself about perimenopause. In fact, it didn't occur to her that her night sweats had anything to do with it. She sought solutions for her night sweats without making the connection. She bought a fan and changed some of the things she ate to keep the night sweats in check so that she could sleep well. As far as she was concerned, perimenopause was a thing for older women. Unfortunately, this assumption meant that she started her journey with little information. She thought perimenopause is a time full of negatives – hot flashes and mood swings.

One night, Ann woke up at around 4am boiling hot. It was as if her internal thermostat broke down in an instant. From then on, heat would come over her with no warning.

Like a flare, like a whoosh, like a furnace. Slowly, she started feeling less like herself. She couldn't articulate it; she just felt out of touch with who she was. Then, a layer of fat seemed to clump around her waist in no time at all. She started feeling invisible. She couldn't work out whether that was real or imagined, but she knew she disliked her new self. She was constantly anxious, grumpy and short tempered.

At 37, the symptoms of perimenopause were too much to bear that they were affecting her daily life. She could barely concentrate at work, and when she finally got 'in the zone,' she would be snapped back by a hot flash. Her periods were irregular and would have her feeling like a teenager, who was just experiencing her first period. After a lot of research and consultation, she got an IUD to manage her periods. She started consulting her gynecologist on the regular. She learnt how to time her alcohol consumption and how to manage stress to fall asleep better. Now, at 45 years of age, Ann finds this stage of life freeing. She doesn't care so much what others think of her. She has a new respect for her body and its ability to transform into what it needs to be.

Christine's Story

When Christine was 45, she started feeling really stressed at work. She was finding it overwhelming and anxiety provoking. She put it down to stress at work because there were a lot of changes happening there. She took a break for a couple of months and returned on a part-time basis working with the person who had covered for her. Then Christine noticed that even though she had only half of her old job, she was still overwhelmed. She had always been good at planning herself, but this time round, she couldn't. Her memory was gone and she constantly felt confused.

Christine started to worry that she had Alzheimer's or dementia. She saw some GPs and they recommended antidepressants even though she didn't really feel depressed.

Eventually she realized that what she was experiencing was perimenopause. She found a group of women online who were sharing their symptoms. She visited a private doctor and he prescribed hormone replacement therapy that ended up solving some of her symptoms but didn't ease the feeling of being overwhelmed. On a number of occasions, she asked for time off from work and had her sick note read 'perimenopause.' Christine says she wants people to know what happened more than she is embarrassed by that.

My Story

For me, the experience of perimenopause came to my consciousness on that fateful day picking up my son from school. I remember a few days having the gray skies cloud my mood; as I explained it to myself. I remember this unshakable sense of fatigue that seemed to wrap itself around me like a heavy, unwelcome cloak.

In the months leading up to that day, I had noticed a growing disquiet in my life. I'd been feeling constantly fatigued and unmotivated, a creeping weariness that lingered even after a full night's sleep. Insomnia had become my unwelcome companion, turning the quiet hours of the night into a restless battleground. At first, I attributed it all to my night shifts—my job required me to work irregular hours, and surely that was the root of my troubles.

Yet, as the weeks passed, I began to suspect there was more to it. My nights were fraught with tossing and turning, and when sleep did come, it was fragmented and unsatisfying. During the day, I found myself struggling to maintain focus and energy. Tasks that once felt routine now seemed insurmountable. It was as if I was wading through life in a thick fog, the vibrant colors of my days turning muted and gray.

The mood swings were perhaps the most bewildering. One moment, I'd be laughing with friends, and the next, a wave of inexplicable sadness or irritability would crash over me, leaving me emotionally drained and perplexed. I tried to rationalize it, attributing it to stress from work or personal life. I kept telling myself that a few more days of rest or a change in routine would set things right.

But despite my efforts to pin down the cause, the symptoms persisted, and the idea that something deeper might be at play started to nag at me. I began to connect the dots between my erratic sleep patterns, mood fluctuations, and persistent fatigue. It was during one of these introspective moments, while I was scanning through articles on women's health, that I first encountered the term "perimenopause." It was as if a light had been turned on in a dark room.

Reading about perimenopause, I found myself nodding along, recognizing the familiar symptoms described. The irregularities, the hot flashes, the sudden waves of fatigue—it all resonated with my experience. The realization was both a relief and a revelation. It wasn't just the night shifts or the stresses of daily life; I was navigating a significant transition in my hormonal landscape.

This newfound understanding didn't immediately resolve the symptoms, but it offered a framework within which I could start addressing them. I began to seek ways to manage my symptoms more effectively, from adjusting my diet to exploring relaxation techniques. It was a process of trial and error, but acknowledging what was happening to my body was the first crucial step in reclaiming some semblance of balance.

In reflecting on that time, I realize how crucial it is to listen to our bodies and seek answers when things feel off. Perimenopause had quietly woven itself into the fabric of my daily life, disrupting it in ways I hadn't initially understood. Now, with a name for the experience, I felt better equipped to navigate this transitional phase with greater awareness and acceptance.

Looking at these four stories, what symptoms did you notice? Do you see how much better the women did after they started learning about their situation? That could be you. I hope that that's you as you read this book.

What Exactly is Perimenopause?

Perimenopause, otherwise called the menopause transition, refers to the period your body begins transitioning to menopause. Throughout this transition period, your ovaries start producing less hormones resulting in an erratic or irregular menstrual cycle.

During perimenopause, your body is moving towards the end of your reproductive years. The transition can begin as early as in your mid-30s to as late as your mid-50s. For some women, the transition is short but for the majority of women, it lasts between four and eight years. In simple terms, perimenopause is the period of your life when it is no longer possible to predict your cycles. Your ovaries start producing less estrogen as you age as they prepare to stop releasing eggs entirely. Your body starts getting ready to lose the ability to get pregnant.

Perimenopause is a natural and normal progression in your reproductive cycle. It happens that as your body adjusts to the different hormone levels, you experience other physical changes and symptoms. During perimenopause, you are experiencing a decline in fertility but it is still possible to become pregnant. It is difficult to say for sure the age your perimenopause will start and the symptoms you will experience because each woman's journey is unique. But you are out of perimenopause once you have had 12 consecutive months without your menstrual period. Essentially, when your periods have ended, you are in menopause.

When Does Perimenopause Occur?

As mentioned earlier, perimenopause can begin as early as a woman's 30s or 40s, although the average age of onset is around 45. However, it's important to note that every woman's experience is unique, and the timing can vary greatly from person to person. Factors such as genetics, lifestyle, and overall health can influence when perimenopause begins.

There are rare cases when a woman enters perimenopause by the age of 30. This means they enter perimenopause at a younger age than the average – early 30s. This is referred to as premature menopause. These women experience symptoms similar to natural menopause, but the causes of premature menopause are unknown. There are some medical procedures or conditions that contribute to premature menopause, though, but when there is no surgical or medical cause for premature menopause, the scientific term for it is primary ovarian insufficiency.

Signs and Symptoms of Perimenopause

While the most apparent sign of perimenopause is irregular periods, there are several other symptoms that women may experience during this phase. This section will break the symptoms down to help you know what you can expect:

1. Changes in menstrual cycle

During perimenopause, periods may become irregular, with variations in flow, duration, and frequency. Some women may experience heavier or lighter bleeding than usual. In the transition period, your body is releasing less of the ovulation hormones hence the changes in your menstrual cycle. Some people also notice significant changes in their premenstrual syndrome symptoms.

One of the most commonly asked questions by women entering perimenopause is how they can know if the changes they are experiencing in their periods are normal perimenopausal changes or something to be worried about. Irregular periods are common during perimenopause, but there can be other conditions contributing to abnormalities in menstrual bleeding. Generally, if any of the following circumstances is true of you, see a healthcare provider to eliminate other causes:

- Your periods are very close together
- Your periods have become very heavy and sometimes have blood clots
- You experience spotting after sex
- You bleed or spot after your period
- Your periods last a number of days more than usual

Abnormal bleeding may be caused by perimenopausal hormonal imbalances, blood-clotting problems, miscarriage, pregnancy-related bleeding, taking blood thinners, endometrial polyps, or fibroids. Consult a medical professional if you are unsure whether the irregularities you are experiencing are due to perimenopause.

Generally, though, if you still get your period, however irregular, you are still ovulated. You have to go for 12 consecutive months without your period to assume you have fully entered menopause.

2. Hot flashes and night sweats

Most women do not expect to experience hot flashes until menopause so it is often a surprise to see them earlier.

Perimenopause is often accompanied by sudden waves of intense heat and sweating. They can occur any time of the day, but are common at night, disrupting sleep. The scientific name for hot flashes is vasomotor symptoms.

Women who experience perimenopause related to a treatment, surgery or some medications tend to struggle more with hot flashes, but they are typical even for natural perimenopause.

Generally, hot flashes come rapidly and last between one and five minutes. Their severity ranges from a feeling of being consumed by fire from within to a fleeting sense of warmth. A major hot flash can induce upper-body and facial flushing, chills, sweating and sometimes confusion. It can be quite disconcerting to have one of these at an inconvenient time like during a job interview or a speech. The frequency of hot flashes varies widely. Some women have a few within a week while other may experience ten or more during the day and some at night.

The physiology of hot flashes has been studied for over three decades, but it is not clear why or how they occur. Most women in the UK and US experience hot flashes during perimenopause, but the experience is different in other parts of the world. Korean, Southeast Asian and Japanese women experience hot flashes far less. In Mexico's Yucatan peninsula, women appear to have very few hot flashes, if at all. These differences are suspected to be tied to lifestyle factors like diet and genetics.

Whatever the case, estrogen is involved in hot flashes, otherwise estrogen therapy would not be able to relieve these symptoms as well as it does. However, estrogen is not the whole story. In one study, researchers found no differences in estrogen levels in women who have no hot flashes versus those who do. More research still needs to be done to understand hot flashes in perimenopause – it could open the way for new non hormonal treatments.

3. Mood swings and irritability

Hormonal fluctuations can impact a woman's emotional well-being, leading to mood swings, irritability, and increased sensitivity. Researchers estimate that between 10 and 20% of women in perimenopause experience mood symptoms. Some studies have linked these mood disruptions to depression, but there is no proof that depression in women during their midlife reflects a change in their hormone levels. Some women actually have lower rates of depression after 45 years of age, than before.

During perimenopause, some women experience changes that make them chronically irritable or anxious. Besides, the unpredictability of perimenopause can be so stressful that it provokes irritability. Typically, some women are more vulnerable to hormone-related changes in their mood than others. How you experience mood changes will be tied to your overall health and mental health history.

4. Sleep disturbances

Many women experience difficulties falling asleep or staying asleep during perimenopause. This can be due to night sweats, anxiety, or other hormonal changes. According to research, 40% of perimenopausal women experience sleep problems.

These sleep problems are mostly tied to the disturbances cause by night sweats – like having to wake up to change sheets during the night – although some are not. The issue of sleep disturbances is often too complex to hinge on hormone fluctuations alone. As we age, sleep cycles are bound to change and insomnia is a common age-related issue for both sexes.

5. Vaginal dryness and discomfort

Decreased estrogen levels can cause vaginal dryness, leading to discomfort during sexual intercourse. This can be explained by the fact that falling estrogen levels cause vaginal tissue to become thinner. Sometimes dryness comes with irritation and itchiness. It can contribute to a decline in sexual desire for some women.

6. Changes in libido

Some women may experience a decrease in sexual desire or changes in their sexual response during perimenopause. It is important to note that these symptoms can vary in severity and duration for each individual. While some women may experience mild symptoms, others may find them more disruptive to their daily lives.

The Role of Hormones During Perimenopause

Your body has been producing estrogen since puberty. Estrogen is produced in your ovaries and plays a vital role in maintaining your reproductive system. During perimenopause, your estrogen levels begin to decline and so the body has to adjust to these changes. When estrogen levels decline, it throws off the balance with progesterone, another hormone produced in the ovaries. Together, these hormones control menstruation and ovulation. Majority of the symptoms you experience are caused by these changing hormone levels. The decrease in estrogen levels can lead to bone thinning and a change in cholesterol levels, for example, which result in physical symptoms like weight gain. By the time you reach menopause, your body produces so little estrogen that the ovaries can no longer release eggs.

Typically, you don't need a healthcare provider to diagnose perimenopause. Most people are able to notice and deal with the changes in their bodies without needing a formal diagnosis, but if you are unsure and experience emotional symptoms that interfere with your ability to function every day, or blood clots in your menstrual discharge, you can consult a healthcare professional.

Healthcare professionals will use your FSH (follicle stimulating hormone) levels to help diagnose perimenopause. FSH is another vital hormone in the reproductive system produced in the pituitary gland – located in the brain. FSH stimulates your ovaries to release the egg during ovulation. When you consult a medical professional, they can test your FSH levels to confirm the start of menopause. Your FSH levels are consistently high during menopause. However, FSH tests can be misleading in perimenopause because your hormones rise and fall erratically. Besides, some medications like hormone therapy or birth control pills affect the results of these hormone tests.

Even so, by the time we get to our late 30s, our bodies do not produce as much progesterone. The amount and quality of follicles also reduce, causing fewer ovulations. As a result, your menstrual flow and cycle length varies. Over time, FSH levels may increase as the body tries to prod the ovaries to produce more estrogen, so a high FSH can be a sign that perimenopause has started.

Understanding perimenopause is the first step in navigating this transitional phase. By recognizing the signs and symptoms, along with the role of hormones, we can gain a better understanding of what to expect during this time of change. With this knowledge, we can seek the support and resources necessary to navigate perimenopause with confidence and grace. In the next chapter, we will go in depth into the physical symptoms of perimenopause to help you know how to navigate them.

Chapter 2
Navigating the Physical Changes

The human body is a complex and finely tuned machine. It is a marvel of biological engineering. Every system within the body is interdependent, operating in a harmonious balance to maintain health and functionality. It relies on the seamless operation of numerous systems, including the cardiovascular, respiratory, digestive, nervous, endocrine, and musculoskeletal systems among others. Each of these systems has subsystems within it and they all perform specialized roles, but do not function in isolation. For example, the cardiovascular system transports oxygen and nutrients supplied by the respiratory and digestive systems to cells throughout the body. The nervous system coordinates these activities, sending signals to regulate heart rate, digestion, and muscle movement. The endocrine system releases hormones that influence almost every function, from growth and metabolism to mood and reproductive health.

When one system thrives, the other systems thrive. On the other hand, when one system encounters an issue or a change, it can trigger a cascade of effects throughout the entire body. A disruption in the endocrine system, for example, can lead to widespread effects. This is particularly evident during perimenopause. During perimenopause, the ovaries gradually produce less estrogen and progesterone, leading to a host of physical and emotional symptoms. In this chapter, you will understand how hormonal changes cause physical symptoms. You will find information to help you understand your menstrual changes at perimenopause. You will learn how to cope with hot flashes and night sweats and you will find tips to maintain a healthy body despite all the changes you are experiencing.

Hormonal Fluctuations

As women, our bodies undergo numerous changes throughout our lives with the major ones being during puberty and perimenopause. Hormones are fundamental to these changes at every stage, from puberty through post-menopause. The Virginia Women's Center describes a hormone as a "chemical communicator or connector" that sends messages between organs in the body. Hormones function like keys that fit into specific locks, or receptor sites, on organs. This inter-organ communication helps maintain balance and optimal function within the body.

At birth, hormone levels are high, but they drop within a few months and stay low until puberty. During puberty, hormonal changes trigger physical transformations in the body. Early in puberty, hormone levels rise, stimulating the production of sex hormones like estrogen. This surge in estrogen leads to the physical changes seen in girls during puberty, including the development of breasts, ovaries, uterus, and vagina, as well as the onset of menstruation.

The average age for the onset of puberty in girls is around ten and a half years old, but it can range from seven to thirteen years. Menarche, or the first menstrual cycle, usually shows up around twelve and a half to thirteen years old. The entire process of puberty typically spans three to four years. For most women, monthly periods continue regularly until perimenopause. All these changes that we experience, can primarily be traced to two hormones: estrogen and progesterone.

Estrogen influences many bodily functions and is essential for the development and maintenance of the reproductive system and secondary sexual characteristics such as body hair and breasts. During puberty, it is estrogen that helps in female sexual development, prompting the growth of breasts, pubic hair, and other sexual characteristics. One of its primary roles is to support the functionality of sexual organs. In the ovaries, estrogen stimulates the growth of the egg follicle. In the vagina, it maintains the thickness of the vaginal wall and plays a role in lubrication. Estrogen also builds up the uterine lining each month, regulates the flow and consistency of uterine mucus secretions, and is crucial for the formation of breast tissue and the cessation of milk production after weaning.

Estrogen is also vital for reproductive health. It controls the growth of the uterine lining at the start of the menstrual cycle and during pregnancy. Beyond its role in the menstrual cycle, estrogen is important for overall health, regulating bone density, cholesterol metabolism, body weight, glucose metabolism, and insulin sensitivity. There are three types of estrogen in the female body: estradiol, estrone, and estriol. Each type plays a different role in reproductive health and their levels fluctuate throughout different life stages. Estrone is the predominant estrogen during perimenopause, while estradiol is most common in women of reproductive age. Generally, when you see a reference to 'estrogen levels' in conversations about perimenopause, it pertains to estradiol, which naturally fluctuates during the menstrual cycle and at perimenopause.

Progesterone, on the other hand, is necessary for preparing the body for pregnancy and supporting it throughout. It is a key hormone in the progestogen class, influencing sexual development and reproduction. It is produced by the ovaries, placenta (during pregnancy), and adrenal glands. The fluctuations of progesterone signal the body to shed the uterine lining, triggering menstruation. The hormone prepares the body for pregnancy in several ways. It readies the uterine lining to receive a fertilized egg, thickens cervical mucus to block harmful bacteria, maintains the uterine lining, and prevents uterine contractions during pregnancy. It also helps prepare the glands and milk ducts for breastfeeding. Progesterone is often used in fertility treatments because it addresses various conditions, including luteal phase deficiency and abnormal uterine bleeding.

If during pregnancy progesterone levels are too low, it can result in early labor or miscarriage. Even so, progesterone is not just useful to our bodies for pregnancy. When your levels become too low, it causes irregular and heavy menstrual bleeding. A lack of progesterone in the bloodstream is often an indication that the ovaries have failed to release an egg during ovulation. During perimenopause, estrogen levels become erratic. They can rise and fall unpredictably, leading to an imbalance. This fluctuation can cause a variety of symptoms such as irregular menstrual cycles, hot flashes, and night sweats. Over time, the overall levels of estrogen decrease as the ovaries produce less of this hormone. This decline contributes to the end of regular menstrual periods and marks the transition to menopause. Lower estrogen levels are responsible for symptoms like vaginal dryness, changes in libido, and mood swings. Estrogen's role in maintaining bone density also means that its decline increases the risk of osteoporosis.

Progesterone levels also decline during perimenopause. This hormone, primarily produced after ovulation, diminishes as ovulation becomes less frequent and eventually stops. The decrease in progesterone can lead to irregular menstrual cycles. Without sufficient progesterone to regulate the cycle, periods can become unpredictable in timing and flow. Lower levels of progesterone can contribute to heavier or lighter periods, increased premenstrual symptoms, and greater fluctuations in mood.

The combined decline and erratic behavior of estrogen and progesterone lead to irregular periods. Women may experience shorter or longer cycles, skipped periods, and varying menstrual flow. The imbalance between estrogen and progesterone also causes a range of physical changes and symptoms, including hot flashes, night sweats, sleep disturbances, anxiety, and depression.

Menstrual Changes

Perimenopause can result in longer periods due to the hormonal fluctuations of estrogen and progesterone. Your menstrual cycle may start earlier or later than usual and can vary in heaviness and duration. During perimenopause, the levels of estrogen and progesterone can vary significantly from month to month. When estrogen levels are higher than progesterone levels, the uterine lining can thicken, causing your body to take longer to shed it, which can lead to longer periods.

If you experience longer periods, it's helpful to keep tampons, pads, or other menstrual supplies on hand so you're always prepared. Track your cycle with a journal or a period-tracking app to help you understand the typical length of your periods and identify any changes. Hormone fluctuations during perimenopause mean each month can be significantly different from the last, resulting in various deviations from your usual cycle. Other menstruation changes you may experience include:

- **Spotting between periods**

Spotting, or bleeding between periods, can occur for several reasons, including changes in birth control. During perimenopause, your cycle becomes unpredictable, and spotting may become more common. While spotting is usually not a cause for concern during this time, it's important to inform your healthcare provider of any excessive bleeding. If your periods are lighter, it is likely due to perimenopause. However, sometimes abnormal bleeding can indicate underlying conditions. Discuss any concerns with your healthcare provider and ensure you keep up with gynecological visits and pelvic exams.

- **Shorter cycles**

Every woman experiences her period uniquely, including variations in cycle length. For many, one of the first signs of perimenopause is a shortening of their menstrual cycles. During perimenopause, hormonal changes cause the follicular phase to shorten, leading to quicker ovulation. This often results in shorter and earlier periods, with cycles sometimes occurring two to three days earlier than expected. It's not uncommon to have two periods within a single month, with another period starting as soon as three weeks after the last one.

If you are concerned about a short and unpredictable cycle, consider using leakage protection like pads, period overwear or liners. Pass on menstrual cups or tampons unless you have your menstrual flow. Insertion can be uncomfortable or difficult without lubrication. You are also very likely to forget to change them, increasing the risk for complications.

- **Missed periods**

Periods can become highly unpredictable during perimenopause, with some women experiencing skipped cycles altogether. After a missed period, it's possible to have an unusually heavy one. The variability in menstrual patterns means that each month can bring different changes. Approximately one in ten women stop menstruating abruptly without prolonged irregularity.

- **Heavier periods**

Heavy bleeding, known as menorrhagia, involves losing 80 mL or more of blood during menstruation. You may be experiencing heavy periods if you frequently soak through tampons or pads. When estrogen levels are higher than progesterone levels, the uterine lining thickens more than usual, resulting in heavier bleeding. While heavy periods are a common symptom of perimenopause, they can pose health risks, including iron deficiency. In rare cases, heavy bleeding may indicate conditions like endometrial cancer or endometrial hyperplasia, where the uterine lining becomes excessively thick due to an overgrowth of cells. Be sure to inform your doctor if you experience heavy periods to rule out serious conditions.

- **Brown or Dark Blood**

Blood can appear dark or brown when it is older and has spent more time in the uterus before being expelled. Fresh blood that exits the body quickly tends to be bright red, which is typical of normal periods. When blood remains in the uterus longer, it becomes oxidized, causing it to darken in color. This can occur during perimenopause, ovulation, or early pregnancy. During perimenopause, it is especially common due to hormonal imbalances. These imbalances cause the uterine lining to break down differently, allowing blood to linger in the uterus longer. If you notice a foul odor with your vaginal discharge, it may be a sign of infection. See your doctor.

Although the likelihood of becoming pregnant during perimenopause decreases, it remains possible. According to the National Center for Health Statistics, there were 840 births among women aged 50 and over in 2017. Additionally, the birth rate for women aged 45 and older was 0.9 births per 1,000 women. This means that if you are in perimenopause and engage in vaginal-penile sex, pregnancy is still a risk.

Track your periods

The changes in your menstrual cycle and the physical symptoms associated with perimenopause can significantly impact daily life. Fortunately, there are strategies to manage these changes and improve comfort during this transition. Before any other strategy, your biggest friend in managing menstrual changes is a journal tracker or a period app. It will provide a clearer understanding of what is happening in your body and the new patterns you can expect.

If your periods come with more pain than before, taking ibuprofen can help with menstrual cramps. Taking ibuprofen while you are heavily bleeding may reduce your flow. In your journal tracker, record other changes that you notice in yourself and track any discomfort or symptoms that you experience. When unsure, consider wearing black underwear or invest in period underwear to prevent staining.

Hot Flashes and Night Sweats

Hot flashes often last for an average of 5 years, and their duration tends to be longer if they start earlier in life. Like the other physical symptoms, hot flashes are caused by fluctuating hormone levels, particularly estrogen and progesterone, which affect the body's temperature regulation. The changes in these hormone levels influence other hormones that control body temperature, leading to sudden feelings of warmth, flushing, and excessive sweating. The frequency and severity of hot flashes and night sweats vary among women. Some may experience occasional hot flashes, while others find that these symptoms significantly disrupt their daily lives.

Nighttime hot flashes, or night sweats, can be particularly troublesome as they cause intense sweating that soaks through sleepwear, waking you up and making it difficult to return to sleep. Hormonal changes affecting body temperature are often more noticeable at night, contributing to these disturbances. While some women adapt to perimenopause-related symptoms, others find them quite disruptive. Doctors often recommend trying lifestyle changes for three months before considering medication.

Some changes that you can try to manage hot flashes include:

- Identify and avoid triggers – Research has identified things like alcohol, spicy foods, caffeine, and smoking as common triggers of hot flashes. Watch the periods you experience them and try to avoid triggers where possible.
- Stay cool - Wear light clothing or when it is cold, dress in layers to easily remove items during a hot flash.
- Use fans - Keep a fan by the bed and maintain a low room temperature with open windows, fans, or air conditioning.

- Take cool showers - Take cool showers during the day and before bed. You can also run cool water over your wrists to quickly cool your body down.
- Maintain a healthy weight - Regular exercise and an active lifestyle can help maintain a healthy weight, which may reduce the frequency and severity of hot flashes.
- Reduce stress - Practice relaxation techniques such as slow, deep breathing and meditation to manage stress and decrease hot flashes.

Weight Gain and Metabolism Changes

Weight gain may seem inevitable as you enter your forties, but it doesn't have to be. Natural hormonal changes can bring symptoms like hot flashes, night sweats, and mood swings, but you shouldn't resign yourself to seeing the number on the scale climb. Here's what's happening with your body when you start gaining weight especially at perimenopause: during perimenopause, weight tends to redistribute, often accumulating around the belly.

As you approach and go through this period, declining estrogen levels and a slowing metabolism make it harder to lose weight, especially around the middle. Belly fat isn't just a nuisance; it's also a health risk. Research published in the journal Menopause indicates that weight gain around the abdomen during perimenopause increases the risk of cardiovascular disease, even if your overall weight hasn't changed. While women tend to gain weight as we age, it's possible to take action against it. It can be hard, but it is possible to do it. To manage weight during this phase, it's important to prioritize a healthy lifestyle that includes regular physical activity, a balanced diet, and strength training exercises to maintain muscle mass.

For exercise, blend moderate and vigorous activities. Try aerobic exercises such as swimming, walking, biking, and jogging, while also incorporating resistance training to build muscle strength. Researchers advise integrating high-intensity interval training (HIIT) into your schedule, alternating between moderate and intense intervals throughout the week. According to the Centers for Disease Control and Prevention (CDC), adults should aim for at least 150 minutes of moderate aerobic activity weekly, along with two or more days of muscle-strengthening exercises targeting major muscle groups. If you opt for HIIT, strive for a balanced mix of moderate and high-intensity workouts each week, in addition to the prescribed strength training sessions.

Bear in mind that our exercise needs evolve as we age. If you find yourself lacking motivation, create incentives to stay active—whether it's closing the rings on your fitness tracker or finding joy in various physical activities. While a gym membership isn't mandatory, you need to maintain muscle strength and rev-up your metabolism through regular strength training. Incorporate exercises that involve lifting, pushing, and pulling to keep your muscles engaged.

While at it, keep your diet balanced. During perimenopause, your metabolism tends to slow down, potentially burning fewer calories each day. Managing calorie intake will help you to prevent excess weight gain during this phase. Besides, because perimenopause often coincides with a shift away from the daily routines of cooking for the family, for some women eating healthy becomes more challenging. After years of cooking, many women opt for dining out, which can lead to consuming excessive calories, particularly when paired with alcohol. To mitigate this, you can try ordering appetizers as main courses and requesting a to-go container for leftovers when indulging in larger meals.

Reduce reliance on restaurant meals and takeout to help in portion control and watch your meal timing and frequency. Contrary to popular belief, emerging research suggests that the traditional approach of eating five or six small meals per day might not be optimal for weight management during perimenopause because your metabolism is slow. Try three square meals a day, starting with a substantial breakfast rich in lean protein and concluding with a lighter supper.

Bone Health

During perimenopause, your body undergoes a decline in estrogen levels. Estrogen, among its many roles, plays a crucial part in maintaining bone density. As estrogen levels decrease, the risk of osteoporosis and bone fractures increases. To safeguard bone health during perimenopause, you need to adopt proactive measures. For starters, you need to ensure an adequate intake of calcium and vitamin D. Calcium is a building block for bones, while vitamin D facilitates calcium absorption, aiding in bone strength.

Incorporating calcium-rich foods like dairy products, leafy greens, and fortified foods into the diet, along with spending time outdoors to promote natural vitamin D synthesis, can help maintain optimal bone health.

Weight-bearing exercises will also help in bone health maintenance during perimenopause. Activities such as walking, jogging, dancing, and strength training exert stress on the bones, stimulating them to become stronger and denser over time. Regular exercise not only helps prevent bone loss but also improves balance and coordination, reducing the risk of falls and fractures.

It's prudent to discuss your bone health concerns with a healthcare professional. This may involve scheduling bone density screenings to assess bone strength and identify any early signs of osteoporosis. Depending on individual risk factors and bone health status, healthcare providers may recommend additional measures such as supplements or medications to support bone density and reduce fracture risk.

Skin and Hair Changes

If you're noticing changes in your hair and skin during perimenopause, the culprit is often the rapid decline in estrogen levels. Estrogen plays a vital role in maintaining skin hydration and plumpness. As estrogen levels decrease, the skin loses some of its moisture-retaining molecules, resulting in dryness. Estrogen also influences hair growth and thickness, so its decline can lead to thinner hair. Perimenopause often brings about noticeable changes in both skin and hair. Here are some of the most common ones:

- **Sagging and decreased plumpness**

Collagen, a key protein responsible for skin structure, declines as estrogen levels drop. This reduction in collagen production results in a loss of skin firmness and elasticity. Some women turn to collagen supplements or collagen-rich foods like bone broth to counteract this effect. Besides those, combatting collagen loss can be as simple as incorporating a nightly facial massage using your preferred moisturizer or facial oil. The massaging action stimulates collagen production in the skin.

- **Dryness, flakiness, and itching**

Perimenopausal skin tends to experience increased dryness, but a consistent home care routine can help manage this issue effectively. Practice gentle cleansing.

Don't let the dry skin dissuade you from cleansing. Cleanse daily to remove impurities. Choose a non-foaming, gentle cleanser designed for sensitive skin. Always moisturize your skin. Moisturizers containing hyaluronic acid help retain moisture, maintaining skin suppleness. Besides, serums and creams with antioxidants, such as vitamin C, combat aging-related free radicals.

Steer clear of products containing fragrance, colorants, or alcohol, as these can exacerbate skin issues. Rather, go for bland, unscented products suitable for sensitive skin. Be sure to optimize your shower habits. Keep showers short and lukewarm, as hot water can strip the skin of its natural oils, leading to dryness. Moisturize immediately after patting dry, as damp skin better absorbs hydration. If you notice redness or rashes, seek advice from a dermatologist. They can assess and address any underlying skin conditions, such as eczema or rosacea, and recommend suitable treatment options.

- **Dark spots**

In perimenopause, those persistent dark marks, often called age spots, tend to make an appearance and can be quite stubborn. Over-the-counter creams may not always be effective against dark spots, but they are a good place to start. Otherwise, go for prescription options like tretinoin, a potent retinoid. Some women also choose, in-office treatments such as facial peels or laser therapies to target individual spots, enhancing overall skin brightness and youthfulness. It's worth discussing these options with your dermatologist.

- **Unwanted facial hair**

As hormonal shifts occur, you might notice unwanted hair cropping up on the upper lip or chin. Traditional methods like tweezing, waxing, hair removal creams, and threading can provide temporary relief. For a more permanent solution, electrolysis offers a viable option. This method destroys hair follicle growth cells, preventing regrowth. Opt for a licensed electrologist or seek recommendations from your doctor. While laser hair removal can effectively eliminate unwanted facial hair, there is a caveat. Laser treatment targets melanin, which dictates hair and skin color. It's most effective on dark hair. Lighter hair may not respond to laser treatment.

- **Perimenopausal acne breakouts**

Not all women experience acne, but some do. Fluctuating hormone levels can lead to acne breakouts. If you're dealing with perimenopause acne, adopt a gentle approach. Many over-the-counter acne products can be overly harsh and drying. Choose a mild cleanser containing salicylic acid. If OTC remedies prove ineffective, seek professional guidance from a dermatologist for prescription solutions.

- **Hair loss and thinning**

Some women may experience hair thinning or shedding because of decreasing estrogen levels during perimenopause. Treat your scalp with care to optimize hair growth. If your scalp is dry, opt for gentle, moisturizing shampoos and reduce washing frequency.

Conversely, oily scalp may benefit from daily shampooing, though individual preferences vary. It is also typical for some women to experience androgenic alopecia, commonly known as female-pattern baldness. Over-the-counter products containing minoxidil can help with this condition. Whatever the case, seek dermatological evaluation if you notice any concerning signs, including distinct bald spots, hair loss accompanied by discomfort, pimple-like bumps along the hairline, excessive hair shedding, or the presence of a rash. Early intervention can help address underlying issues effectively.

Prioritize sun protection

Regardless of your skin concerns, sunscreen should be a non-negotiable part of your daily routine. Apply it generously every day, throughout the year, to shield your skin from the harmful effects of the sun, which can accelerate aging and increase the risk of skin cancer. Choose a broad-spectrum sunscreen with an SPF of 30 or higher. Selecting one that you enjoy using will increase the likelihood of consistency each morning. When spending time outdoors, remember to reapply every two hours or after swimming, sweating, or drying off with a towel. The sun's rays can prematurely age your skin and heighten the risk of skin cancer. Even during winter months, UV rays can penetrate through clouds.

Breast Health

Breast health becomes increasingly important during perimenopause as hormonal fluctuations can induce changes in breast tissue. You need to be watchful about your breast health to notice any unusual changes. One of the most effective ways to monitor breast health is through regular breast self-examinations. Familiarize yourself with the typical look and feel of your breasts. That way, you can quickly detect any changes or abnormalities. Healthcare professionals often recommend performing self-exams monthly, ideally a few days after the end of menstruation when breasts are less likely to be swollen or tender.

Mammograms play a vital role in breast health maintenance during perimenopause. Schedule a mammogram regularly. These screening tests can detect abnormalities such as lumps or calcifications that may indicate the presence of breast cancer. Healthcare providers typically recommend mammograms at regular intervals, with the frequency determined by factors such as age, family history, and personal risk factors. Give prompt medical attention if any changes or concerns regarding breast health arise. Whether you discover a new lump, notice changes in breast size or shape, experience nipple discharge, or any other unusual symptoms. Early detection and intervention significantly improve the chances of successful treatment and favorable outcomes.

Perimenopause encompasses many physical changes, each influenced by hormonal fluctuations within the body and each combination of symptoms different for every woman. By acknowledging the multifaceted nature of these transformations—ranging from menstrual irregularities to bone health concerns—and actively addressing them, we can reclaim agency over our physical well-being and make the transition much less bothersome.

Through a combination of self-awareness and proactive measures, such as regular self-examinations and screenings, we can mitigate potential health risks and optimize our overall health outcomes. In the next chapter you will learn more about the emotional symptoms associated with perimenopause and find tips on how to manage them.

Chapter 3:
The Emotional Rollercoaster During Perimenopause

The human mind is complex. This is particularly evident in our emotional intelligence—the ability to perceive, manage, and express emotions, as well as recognize them in others. Hormones play a pivotal role in mental health. They exert a profound influence on our emotional states and behaviors. A deeper understanding of this connection holds the potential to enhance emotional well-being significantly. This understanding is especially pertinent for women grappling with emotional distress stemming from hormonal imbalances, such as those associated with conditions like polycystic ovary syndrome (PCOS), endometriosis, premenstrual syndrome (PMS), and for our case, perimenopause. In most cases, you can address hormonal imbalances through simple lifestyle adjustments, but that has to begin with understanding. That's what this chapter is for: to give you the knowledge to empower you to manage your emotional states better.

Hormonal Impact on Emotions

When a girl reaches puberty, her ovaries start releasing estrogen every month along with her menstrual cycle. Around the middle of the cycle, estrogen levels go up quickly, which causes an egg to be released (ovulation). Then, they drop just as fast. For the rest of the month, estrogen levels go up and down more slowly. Normal estrogen levels can be very different from one day to another for the same person, or between two women on the same day of their cycle. But even if we measure estrogen levels, it doesn't tell us much about how someone might be feeling emotionally.

But estrogen does have a big role in controlling our moods. It doesn't just affect our bodies, it also affects parts of our brains that control how we feel. Here are some things estrogen does:

- It helps increase serotonin levels in our brains, which makes us feel happier.
- It changes how endorphins, (chemicals that make us feel good,) work in our brains.
- It also helps protect our nerves and might help them grow.

But even though estrogen seems to have these good effects on the brain, some women actually feel better emotionally after they've gone through menopause, when their estrogen levels are very low. Some experts think that some women are more sensitive to the ups and downs of estrogen during their menstrual cycles. They believe it's these hormone changes during the years when women can have babies that can make some women feel moody. So, do hormones control our emotions?

Yes, it's true that many women go through big changes in how they feel and act at different times in their lives, like when they start puberty, have a baby, or go through perimenopause and menopause. Since all of these changes are caused by hormones, it makes sense to think that hormones are closely connected to our emotions. But it's not as simple as saying 'this hormone equals this emotion.' There are lots of different ways we can feel emotions, which makes things more complicated.

Sometimes, something specific can make us feel an emotion. For example, just seeing an ice cream van could trigger lots of different feelings: you might feel happy because you love ice cream, or you might really want some ice cream, or you might even feel jealous that other people are getting ice cream and you're not. Here's a simple diagram to explain what happens in our bodies when something triggers an emotion:

The trigger - Something sets off one of our senses.

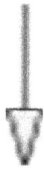

↓

Memory kicks in - The trigger makes the part of our brain that remembers things think about past experiences related to what our senses are telling us.

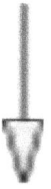

↓

Neurotransmitters (like serotonin and dopamine) send this information to the pituitary gland.

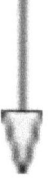

↓

The pituitary gland tells the endocrine glands to change hormone levels, either up or down.

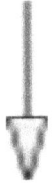

These changes in hormone levels cause physical and emotional reactions. For example, seeing the ice cream van might make you really want some ice cream (an emotional reaction) and start to make you drool (a physical reaction).

But sometimes, there doesn't have to be a clear reason for why we feel emotions. This is especially true for people who have depression but can't explain why. There are lots of ideas about why this happens, like chemical imbalances, problems with how the brain regulates moods, or genetic factors.

Neurotransmitters not only signal the endocrine system to release hormones, but hormones also have the power to regulate neurotransmitters. This is the relationship that is in play when you have hormonal imbalance. When sex hormones are balanced, estrogen boosts serotonin and dopamine activity in the brain, promoting feelings of happiness and motivation. Similarly, optimal levels of testosterone contribute to enhanced dopamine activity. Progesterone closely interacts with neurotransmitters like GABA, which promotes calmness and contentment when balanced, and glutamate, which supports mental alertness and contentment.

Imbalances in these hormones disrupt neurotransmitter function, leading to emotional turmoil characterized by feelings of sadness, lack of motivation, anxiety, and other negative emotions. Such imbalances may also manifest in certain behaviors, such as decreased activity, social withdrawal, increased snacking, and alcohol consumption.

During perimenopause, estrogen levels fluctuate irregularly and can be quite unpredictable. They cause a lot of emotional changes. For example, up to 10% of women may experience depression, which is linked to these unstable estrogen levels. Since hormonal fluctuations, particularly the decline in estrogen, can have a profound impact on a woman's mood and emotional well-being, understanding these changes can help women navigate the emotional rollercoaster more effectively.

Mood Swings and Irritability

Studies have revealed that approximately 23 percent of women will experience mood swings during perimenopause. Some women may encounter intense mood swings, along with feelings of anxiety and depression. The mood swings during perimenopause tend to be quite extreme, catching women off guard and feeling more intense than any previous mood swings. Many of my friends going through perimenopause describe feeling overwhelmed or like they're losing control. They find it challenging to maintain their usual routines as they feel exhausted, emotional, and even forgetful at times. The changes during this period of life affect almost every aspect of a woman's life, with mood swings often being the most difficult aspect to cope with.

Mood swings during perimenopause can be tied to a number of factors. For starters estrogen, the primary female sex hormone, plays a crucial role in regulating mood by affecting serotonin levels in the body. As estrogen levels decline during perimenopause, serotonin levels may also decrease, leading to feelings of depression and increased emotional sensitivity. Progesterone also begins to decline during perimenopause. As progesterone levels drop, estrogen may become dominant, contributing to irritability and feelings of depression. Progesterone helps calm the brain and promotes sleep, so a decrease in progesterone levels can disrupt sleep patterns and contribute to feelings of anxiety.

Mood swings are also tied to hormonal fluctuations. These fluctuations can be unpredictable and destabilizing. Estrogen levels may fluctuate erratically, leading to sudden surges or drops in hormone levels, particularly noticeable in the second half of the menstrual cycle. Perimenopause disrupts the delicate balance of hormones in the body, with reductions and fluctuations affecting mood. It doesn't help that you are likely not sleeping enough. Sleep disruptions are common during perimenopause, primarily due to changes in estrogen and progesterone levels and the associated hot flashes and night sweats, disrupting sleep patterns and exacerbating feelings of anxiety.

Imagine all these changes coupled with the pressures of life and you understand why you get irritable. Many women experience significant life pressures during perimenopause, such as caring for children and aging parents, maintaining a career, and dealing with other responsibilities. It also happens that perimenopause marks the end of the childbearing years for many women, which can be a difficult realization, especially for those who have fertility issues or unresolved desires regarding children. Top that off with the "empty nest" phenomenon and you have a woman overwhelmed by feelings of distress and anxiety.

Perimenopausal mood swings can be severe, but when you remember that they are often driven by significant physical changes in the body, you can begin to manage them.

Seeking therapeutic approaches like cognitive-behavioral therapy (CBT) or hypnotherapy can help manage symptoms and provide support alongside conventional medical treatments. Besides, you also need to:

- **Address stress**

Persistent stress can have detrimental effects on both your mental and physical well-being. As we enter perimenopause, we will often face heightened stress levels due to various life changes, such as career shifts, disrupted sleep, parenting challenges, caring for aging parents, and relationship issues. This accumulation of stressors can increase vulnerability to infections and depression, going by research conducted by the North American Menopause Society (NAMS). Life stressors contribute to irritability across all age groups, with the hormonal fluctuations during perimenopause intensifying their impact. Implement relaxation techniques like deep breathing and meditation to get some relief.

- **Lean on your support systems**

During perimenopause, seeking support from friends and trusted partners can be invaluable. Social connections have a major role in navigating perimenopause. Maintain an active social life. Having friends with whom to share experiences can provide comfort and understanding. Consider joining a local or online support group to connect with others going through similar experiences. Research published in December 2022 underscores the benefits of open discussions about menopausal and perimenopausal experiences, enhancing awareness, reducing barriers to seeking assistance, and ultimately improving care during this universal transition.

Anxiety and Depression

I have learned that Perimenopause can also increase the risk of anxiety and depression. Hormonal imbalances, combined with other factors such as life transitions or personal stressors, can contribute to these mental health challenges. Let me paint for you a picture with a story about a woman. I'll call her Teri. She was in her mid-40s when she started noticing changes in her body. Her symptoms were regular perimenopausal symptoms but she didn't have the knowledge to recognize them. For example, her period became irregular and more intense. She started having hot flashes, put on weight and her energy levels were at an all time low so she stopped doing things she loved like solo travel.

At the time, Teri was working remotely, a lifestyle that didn't help her when she started withdrawing from friends. She felt isolated and unmoored. There was a constant fog over her and she felt like she couldn't find solid ground. Teri didn't know that hormonal changes associated with perimenopause were causing her the feelings of depression and anxiety she was experiencing. As a younger woman, she had a diagnosis of major depression so she figured it was just another one of those. She started having suicidal thoughts and feeling completely hopeless.

Fortunately, when she had the foresight to consult a doctor for depression, the doctor had the foresight to suggest that Teri manage perimenopausal symptoms before taking antidepressants. It worked for her. She started feeling less sluggish and sad. It is common to feel like you have PMS all the time during perimenopause. You don't feel like you are in control of your life. According to research, 18% of women in early perimenopause and 38% of women in late perimenopause experience depression. They also report anxiety symptoms such as panic attacks. The women with a history of mental illness tend to be most at risk and particularly sensitive to the hormonal fluctuations of perimenopause.

In Teri's case, at least she was familiar with depression so she knew to seek help. She had been depressed several times before and had proactively sought treatment. She knew how to advocate for herself. She knew how to recognize her triggers and symptoms. In some cases, though, women are experiencing anxiety and depression for the first time during perimenopause and they don't even know to look for them. They concentrate so much on physical changes that they miss the symptoms of depression. The physical nature of perimenopause can be consuming. It doesn't help that some doctors do not offer tips for those symptoms.

Most physicians, even GP's, get very little education about perimenopause, which is why empowering yourself with information is a good idea so that you can advocate for yourself. Be direct with your doctor about your mental health symptoms the same way you would be direct if you had a rash. That way, you will avoid going years without realizing that you are depressed. It is also a good idea to get counseling. You don't have to cope with everything on your own. You owe it to yourself and to the people around you that you aren't suffering.

So, if feelings of persistent sadness or disinterest persist for more than two weeks, seek the guidance of a therapist. This is based on the perimenopausal guidelines outlined in the Journal of Women's Health. You can also consider cognitive behavioral therapy (CBT) to manage your mood and alleviate depressive symptoms during this transition. CBT helps you reframe your thoughts about your experiences. It addresses the underlying psychological issues behind depression. It would also teach you how to self-advocate with your loved ones. I have found that communication is key here. Simple things like letting your loved ones know how you are feeling. For example, just explaining to others 'I don't feel ready to talk right now, please give me some space' makes a big difference. I have also found it is crucial to avoid getting myself in situations that will heighten emotions like anger, anxiety, fear as these types of emotions hold a detrimental effect on your mental health. Counseling helps manage them.

Brain Fog

Brain fog is a common symptom associated with perimenopause. This term describes difficulties with memory, concentration, and focus. During perimenopause, fluctuating levels of estrogen and progesterone can impact brain function. Estrogen, in particular, is vital for maintaining healthy brain cells and their connections. As estrogen levels decrease, symptoms of brain fog may become more noticeable.

Research indicates that women in perimenopause often report cognitive difficulties such as:

- Forgetfulness
- Trouble focusing
- Memory lapses
- Slower information processing

Because sleep disturbances are common during perimenopause they worsen brain fog symptoms. Poor quality or insufficient sleep can negatively affect cognitive function and memory.

Brain fog often manifests as forgetfulness. I've had my share of these moments, and let me tell you, they can be both disorienting and alarming.

For example, there was a day when I went grocery shopping on my day off. I paid using contactless, so I didn't need to enter my PIN. Later, I went to fill up my car with gas. I tried to pay with my card using contactless again, but this time, it was rejected and asked for my PIN. To my dismay, I couldn't recall what it was! I attempted to enter it three times before my card was blocked. I felt a surge of panic and embarrassment, especially when I had to call my husband to get the PIN, only to find out it was too late. Luckily, my colleague, covered the payment, and I repaid her later. Despite the practical resolution, the experience left me in tears, overwhelmed by the sudden and inexplicable lapse in memory.

Another instance happened at work. I had driven with my colleagues to an off-site meeting. On the way back, a bright, sunny day was marred by an intense hot flush. I cranked up the air conditioning, trying to cool down, but then the road was unexpectedly closed. I followed the diversion, and despite being very familiar with the area, I found myself disoriented. I could see landmarks I recognized, but I couldn't remember where to turn. Embarrassed and anxious, I kept driving around, trying to find our workplace without admitting I was lost. For almost 15 minutes, I circled around, my anxiety mounting with each passing moment. Eventually, a colleague noticed my distress and asked where we were headed. With tears in my eyes, I confessed that I was lost. She guided me back, but the experience left me feeling both frustrated and anxious, questioning my mental sharpness.

In response to these challenges, I decided to take proactive steps to combat brain fog. I rediscovered my love for reading, immersing myself in books to keep my mind engaged and vibrant. I also started taking online courses, which have been excellent for enhancing cognitive function and reducing forgetfulness. Practicing mindfulness has become a crucial part of my daily routine, allowing me to center myself and reduce stress before bed.

Effective time management and early planning have also become vital in my life. By organizing my schedule well in advance, I've found that I can avoid the anxiety and stress that often trigger brain fog. This approach has helped me stay calm and focused, whether I'm preparing for travel or tackling work projects.

While perimenopause certainly brings its share of challenges, these strategies have helped me regain a sense of control and clarity. And though moments of brain fog can still occur, I'm learning to navigate them with greater resilience and understanding.

As a thing to note, although hormone replacement therapy (HRT) is not typically prescribed solely for brain fog, it may address other perimenopausal symptoms. Other lifestyle adjustments can help mitigate brain fog, including:

- Consuming a balanced diet rich in omega-3 fatty acids and antioxidants
- Engaging in regular physical activity, such as yoga or walking
- Incorporating stress management practices, like meditation or deep breathing exercises
- Ensuring adequate sleep (7-8 hours per night)

Additionally, cognitive training and memory exercises can be beneficial in enhancing mental clarity.

It's important to remember that brain fog is usually a temporary condition, with symptoms often improving after later in life. If you experience persistent or severe brain fog, it's advisable to consult with your healthcare provider to rule out other potential issues and develop a tailored management plan.

Self-Care and Stress Management

Let me begin this section by sharing three stories of women, what self-care did for them and what it has come to mean.

Laura Roberts

Laura Roberts had always been the anchor in her family's life. From nurturing her children to supporting her spouse, and even caring for her aging parents, she was the glue that held everyone together. Yet, as Laura entered perimenopause, she realized that she had neglected one important aspect of her life—herself.

For Laura, self-care became an essential part of navigating this new phase. She understood that she needed to shift her focus from being a constant caregiver to taking care of her own physical, emotional, and spiritual needs. She began with small, manageable changes. Every day, she carved out ten minutes for meditation and journaling, which helped her center herself and process her emotions. She also started paying more attention to her diet, opting for organic foods to nourish her body during this time of change.

Laura noticed that her skin was becoming increasingly dry, so she made it a habit to apply moisturizer after every shower. She also found that her sleep patterns were disrupted, so she allowed herself the luxury of an afternoon rest with a good book, and occasionally took short naps to recharge.

One of the more significant steps Laura took was to address her mental health. She spoke openly with her doctor about the depression she was experiencing due to hormonal shifts and began a course of antidepressants. This decision was a pivotal part of her self-care routine and made a profound difference in her overall well-being.

Laura's approach to self-care was a journey of rediscovery, allowing her to manage the challenges of perimenopause with grace and resilience.

Emily Carter

For Emily Carter, self-care during peri-menopause was about embracing a new chapter of life with intention and self-awareness. Understanding the impact of perimenopause on her body, Emily focused on making dietary changes and prioritizing sleep. She knew that these were crucial to maintaining her health and managing stress during this transitional period.

But beyond diet and sleep, Emily discovered that self-care also meant asserting her own needs. She learned to give herself permission to step away from the demands of her family without guilt. If she needed a moment of solitude, she took it, knowing that it was essential for her well-being. Emily became skilled at setting boundaries and saying no to requests that added unnecessary stress to her life. This newfound confidence in her ability to prioritize herself was liberating.

Emily's journey through perimenopause also brought her to a realization about the nature of this life stage. She embraced it not as a permanent state of discomfort but as a transition that would eventually lead to a renewed sense of self. Though it was sometimes challenging, she found that perimenopausal life offered a new sense of freedom—freedom to care for herself without apologies.

My Self-Care practices

For me, self-care looks like a number of activities that nurture both my mind and body, offering a balance between indulgence and discipline.

One of my favorite self-care rituals is cooking. I take immense joy in preparing meals, and cooking has become a true form of escapism for me. Whether I'm crafting elaborate dishes for a crowd or simply experimenting with new recipes, being in the kitchen is my personal adventure. My culinary creativity flows freely when I'm alone with my trusty Alexa speaker, which plays my favorite tunes and keeps me company. Cooking not only allows me to explore my passion for food but also provides a soothing retreat into my own world.

I also practice gratitude daily, starting and ending each day with a moment of prayer and reflection. This ritual helps me maintain a positive outlook and appreciate the small joys in life.

A good night's sleep is crucial for my well-being, and I've found that sipping on herbal teas helps if I ever struggle to fall asleep. Staying well-hydrated is another cornerstone of my self-care routine. I make sure to drink at least two liters of water each day, steering clear of fizzy drinks and sugary juices. Additionally, I've embraced cold showers in the morning, which invigorate me and promote healthy blood circulation.

When it comes to skincare, I use all-natural lotions from Holland and Barrett, particularly those with royal jelly, which I've found to have excellent anti-aging properties.

As someone who has always loved wearing high heels, I've adapted to changes in my body over time. While I still enjoy wearing heels, I've moved away from the six-inch stilettos of my younger years. My goal is to continue wearing stylish heels comfortably well into my seventies.

Maintaining a vibrant social life is important to me, but I've also learned the value of solitude. Time alone allows me to listen to my inner voice, reflect, and plan for the future. To relax and unwind, I regularly indulge in deep tissue massages, including Thai and Indian head massages, often sharing these experiences with my Jamaican mum.

These sessions help ease tension and restore balance to both body and mind.

Finally, I take daily multivitamins, specifically the Well Woman brand by Vitabiotics. Despite my efforts to eat a balanced diet, I know that not all vitamins and nutrients are absorbed efficiently. These supplements provide a valuable backup, ensuring that my body receives the support it needs.

In weaving together these practices, I create a self-care routine that nourishes me physically, mentally, and emotionally, helping me navigate life's challenges with grace and resilience. I will talk about different aspects that inform my self-care practices in different chapters. For example, diet will be in Chapter 5. I talk about different herbs you can try in Chapter 7. The idea is to provide you the information to use to tailor to yourself.

You will notice that self-care looks different for everyone. The essence of self-care is to meet your own needs, and since those are unique, your self-care routine also needs to be unique.

During perimenopause, prioritizing self-care and stress management is crucial for maintaining emotional well-being and navigating the challenges you experience. Engage in activities that bring joy and relaxation, such as hobbies, exercise, or spending time with loved ones. It can play a pivotal role in reducing stress levels and promoting overall mental health. Some self-care practices you can embody include:

- **Take up a hobby**

Hobbies such as painting, gardening, or playing a musical instrument can provide a welcome escape from the stresses of daily life and offer a sense of accomplishment. Immersing yourself in activities that resonate with your personal interests and passions, helps you cultivate a sense of purpose and satisfaction that contributes to emotional well-being.

- **Get moving**

Regular exercise is another essential component of self-care during perimenopause. Physical activity not only helps maintain overall health and fitness but also serves as a powerful stress-reliever. Whether it's going for a brisk walk, practicing yoga, or participating in a dance class, exercise releases endorphins – the body's natural mood lifters – and can help alleviate symptoms of anxiety and depression. Additionally, the social aspect of group fitness activities can provide valuable social support and camaraderie, further enhancing emotional resilience.

- **Spend time with your loved ones**

Spending quality time with loved ones is another effective way to manage stress and foster emotional well-being during perimenopause. Whether it's sharing a meal with family members, catching up with friends over coffee, or simply enjoying a leisurely stroll with a partner, meaningful connections with others can provide comfort, support, and a sense of belonging. These interpersonal relationships serve as a source of strength and encouragement during the challenging days.

- **Practice mindfulness**

Practicing mindfulness techniques can be immensely beneficial for managing emotional fluctuations during perimenopause. Mindfulness is about cultivating present-moment awareness and non-judgmental acceptance of your thoughts, feelings, and bodily sensations. Techniques such as meditation, deep breathing exercises, and progressive muscle relaxation can help calm the mind, reduce stress levels, and promote a greater sense of inner peace and balance.

- **Adopt a nutrient-rich diet**

Ensuring your diet is rich in essential nutrients can contribute to hormone balance, reduce inflammation, manage weight, alleviate hot flashes, and support bone health. A nutrient-rich diet encompasses a variety of fruits, vegetables, legumes, whole grains, lean proteins, and healthy fats. It's also important to practice portion control and limit intake of processed foods, excessive salt, spicy foods, added sugars, and caffeine.

- **Prioritize quality sleep**

Good sleep habits are essential for overall well-being. They include maintaining a consistent sleep schedule, engaging in a calming bedtime routine, and creating a cool and comfortable sleep environment. Avoid consuming caffeine, nicotine, and alcohol close to bedtime (at least four to six hours prior) to promote better sleep quality. You can also wear moisture-wicking sleepwear and use breathable bedding to mitigate discomfort associated with night sweats.

It is not enough to manage your physical symptoms, you have to pay attention to your mental health too. By prioritizing self-care and stress management strategies during perimenopause, you can empower yourself to navigate this transitional phase with greater resilience and emotional well-being.

Communication and Support

While perimenopause is a natural and inevitable stage of life, the emotional challenges it presents can often feel overwhelming. Open and honest communication with loved ones can make a significant difference in navigating these challenges and fostering a sense of understanding and support.

Personally, I had to sit down with my husband and our two sons—one grown and one still navigating the turbulent seas of adolescence—to share my experiences and the impact these changes have on me.

I explained that perimenopause brings with it moments of intense overwhelm, during which I might find myself unable to engage in meaningful conversations or offer the attentive listening that I usually strive for. I emphasized that while these moments are not frequent, they are genuine and affect my ability to interact as I would like. When I find myself in such a state, I've learned to voice my needs clearly: "I really can't talk right now, but when I am ready to engage or listen effectively, I'll let you know."

Initially, my adult son seemed to grasp this with a mature understanding. He recognized that my need for space wasn't a reflection of my feelings towards him but rather a necessary step for my own well-being. His supportive response and patience have been a comforting constant.

My teenage son, on the other hand, faced a more challenging adjustment. His eagerness to discuss everything from his latest interests to his daily dilemmas often met with my need for solitude. At first, he interpreted my pauses and temporary withdrawals as rejection - a painful misunderstanding that could have strained our interactions.

However, over time and with continued explanations, he began to see my need for space not as a dismissal of his thoughts but as a response to the unpredictable nature of hot flashes and emotional surges that come with perimenopause.

Hot flashes can strike anytime—whether I'm out in the sun or absorbed in the mundane task of cooking. They are relentless and indifferent to my schedule or the conversations I'm trying to maintain. In those moments, my body's sudden heat clouds my capacity to engage. My sons have started to understand that when I need a moment, it's a chance for all of us to pause and regroup rather than a rejection of their need for connection.

We are still learning to communicate with each other and adjust to each other's needs, but I am grateful I had that conversation with them. Now I don't have to handle the extra layer of their demands on me at a moment when I don't have the capacity to meet them.

One of the most effective ways to navigate the emotional challenges of perimenopause is through open and honest communication with partners, family members, and friends.

By explaining the hormonal changes occurring during perimenopause and their impact on emotions, you can help your loved ones better understand the challenges you are facing. You provide them insight into the physical and emotional symptoms of perimenopause, and empower them to offer empathy, compassion, and practical assistance.

Do not feel shy. It is okay to openly discuss topics such as mood swings, irritability, anxiety, and depression. That way, you can dispel misconceptions and myths surrounding perimenopause. Education and awareness about the hormonal fluctuations that occur at perimenopause can foster greater empathy and understanding among loved ones. Partners, family members, and friends who are informed about the emotional challenges you are experiencing are better equipped to provide the necessary support and encouragement.

You can also consider joining support groups or online communities of women going through perimenopause. It can offer a valuable source of camaraderie and empathy. Connecting with others who are experiencing similar challenges provides a sense of validation and reassurance. You get to share experiences, exchange advice, and offer support within these communities which can foster a sense of solidarity and empowerment.

Support groups and online communities create a safe and nurturing space for us to express our thoughts, feelings, and concerns openly. Whether meeting in person or connecting virtually, these networks offer a platform for women to seek guidance, share coping strategies, and receive validation from peers who understand the unique challenges of perimenopause.

The emotional rollercoaster during perimenopause can be challenging, but by understanding the hormonal impact on emotions and implementing self-care strategies, you can navigate this phase with resilience and grace. Seeking support from loved ones, practicing stress management techniques, and being open to professional help when needed are essential steps in maintaining emotional well-being. Remember, you are not alone on this journey, and with the right tools and support, you can embrace the emotional changes and emerge stronger on the other side. In the next chapter, you will learn how to nurture your relationships despite everything you are going through so that you guarantee yourself a healthy support system.

Chapter 4
Nurturing Relationships During Perimenopause

One of the reasons why I have a chapter on nurturing relationships is because during perimenopause, you need your relationships to thrive so that they can help you thrive. And yet, the very nature of perimenopause can cause relationship problems because it impacts how you feel and act around others. This chapter will help you understand how perimenopause can affect different types of relationships and what to do about it:

Your Relationship With Yourself

Whether in perimenopause or not, the relationship you have with yourself forms the foundation for the relationships with others. It informs how you love, give, influence and care for others. A great relationship with yourself means a higher likelihood of developing greater relationships with others. It follows that nurturing the relationship with yourself is the first step to nurturing relationships with others during perimenopause.

I recall a pivotal moment of clarity when I sat with myself, confronting the reality of the changes that perimenopause had ushered into my life. The initial reaction was one of resistance—grappling with the fear of aging and feeling less attractive. But as I allowed myself to truly accept these changes, I discovered a new pathway forward. Acceptance became my ally, dissolving the inner conflicts that arose from my anxieties about growing older. It was through this acceptance that I could chart a course for the future, free from the shackles of self-rejection.

With acceptance came empowerment. I realized that I no longer needed to adhere to old expectations or pressures. Instead, I could make choices that were genuine and aligned with my authentic self. For instance, I began to prioritize activities that brought me joy when I felt ready, without succumbing to external pressures or guilt. This autonomy over my choices allowed me to engage in self-care practices that resonated deeply with me.

One of the most cherished rituals I embraced was dedicating time to self-love and care. Early morning swims became my sanctuary, where the water's embrace invigorated both my body and spirit. The serene walks by the river, with the soothing sound of flowing water, provide a tranquil space for reflection and relaxation. These moments of solitude are not merely escapes but transformative experiences that calm my mind and nurture my soul.

Traveling has also become another profound source of joy. The world's beauty captivates me, and I set out on a mission to explore as many countries as possible. Each journey gives new perspectives and experiences, enriching my life and reinforcing my sense of self. The act of immersing myself in different cultures and landscapes deepens my appreciation for life's vast tapestry, adding layers of fulfillment to my inner world.

Maintaining healthy and meaningful friendships has also been a cornerstone of my journey. Many of my friends are of similar age or older, and these relationships provide invaluable support and perspective. The shared experiences and wisdom we exchange help anchor me during times of change, reminding me that I am not alone in this process.

Self-acceptance will always ripple outward and enhance your connections with others. By fostering a compassionate and supportive inner dialogue, I've been able to extend that same kindness and understanding to those around me. The strength of my relationships with my family and friends has grown, reflecting the harmony I've cultivated within myself. I've found that the path to nurturing relationships with others becomes clearer and more fulfilling. Self-love and acceptance equip us to love, support, and connect with the people in our lives.

Communication with Loved Ones

Perimenopausal mood swings can significantly impact our interactions with friends. One moment, we may feel perfectly fine, but the next, we might become irritable or angry without warning. It can be challenging for our friends to understand these sudden shifts in mood, especially when they occur during what should be enjoyable social outings. Top that off with social anxiety which can emerge during menopause and you have the perfect storm. Anxiety causes discomfort in group settings or crowded environments. The prospect of being in situations with loud music and numerous people can trigger feelings of unease and reluctance to participate in social activities, so you begin to act differently around your friends.

Not only that, declining confidence, often influenced by hormonal changes and shifts in body image, can affect our friendships. Weight gain or changes in appearance may lead to feelings of self-consciousness and alienation from friends who appear unaffected by similar issues. We become afraid about criticism of our appearance or perceived inadequacies which further diminishes our confidence and willingness to engage socially. Poor sleep quality can further exacerbate these challenges, leaving us feeling fatigued and disinclined to participate in social gatherings or outings. Nights disrupted by night sweats or frequent trips to the bathroom can leave us craving rest and solitude rather than social interaction.

Our romantic relationships are also affected. One recurring concern about romantic relationships revolves around explaining our feelings to our partners without sparking arguments. Many women struggle to convey their emotions effectively, leading to a sense of helplessness. Perimenopause is an emotional rollercoaster, from fleeting moments of anger or irritability to prolonged periods of anxiety and low mood. It's challenging for partners to understand these shifts, especially if they've known us as calm and collected people.

Communication is key here. Find a moment away from home, perhaps during a walk or a meal, to express how you're feeling and how hormonal changes are intensifying your emotional experiences. While your partner may not fully grasp the intricacies of your experience, they can still offer support and comfort. Sometimes, a simple hug or a cup of tea can make a world of difference in defusing tension and breaking the cycle of irritability and anger.

If verbal communication feels daunting, consider sharing resources like this book on peri-menopause. Many women have found that providing educational materials to their partners helps them gain a deeper understanding of the challenges faced during this phase of life. It's heartening to hear feedback from women whose partners have become more empathetic and supportive after reading such resources. Despite these hurdles, maintaining friendships during peri-menopause remains essential for our well-being. Friends can provide invaluable support and understanding during perimenopause, offering a sense of companionship and empathy that may be lacking in other areas of our lives.

As a side note, not all friendships are beneficial during Peri-menopause. Toxic or unsupportive friends can exacerbate feelings of isolation and dissatisfaction, leaving us questioning the value of these relationships. Friends who monopolize conversations or dismiss our struggles can further contribute to feelings of alienation and loneliness.

Comparisons with other Peri-menopause friends who may have fewer symptoms or difficulties can intensify feelings of inadequacy and isolation. It's crucial to recognize the importance of supportive friendships while also acknowledging when certain relationships may be detrimental to our well-being. Navigating friendships during Peri-menopause requires understanding, patience, and a willingness to prioritize self-care and healthy boundaries.

Explaining Changes in Libido and Intimacy

Perimenopause often stirs up questions and challenges that many women grapple with. Some of the common concerns and questions surrounding how menopause affects our romantic connections include:

- **I feel like I am falling out of love**

One pressing issue that often arises is whether menopause can make us feel like we're falling out of love. Surprisingly, the answer is yes. The hormone oxytocin, often dubbed the "cuddle hormone" or "love hormone," plays a significant role in fostering feelings of love and affection. However, as estrogen levels decline during menopause, so does oxytocin production. This hormonal shift can lead to a noticeable decrease in feelings of love and connection with our partners. Some women may suddenly find themselves questioning the strength of their relationship or viewing their partner in a different light.

It's crucial not to rush into any decisions based solely on these feelings. Many women have reported experiencing a resurgence of affection and attachment once their hormonal fluctuations stabilize. Take the time to reflect and communicate openly with your partner. It will help navigate this challenging phase with greater clarity and understanding.

- **I don't desire sex but my partner doesn't get it**

Another common issue revolves around changes in libido and sexual desire. As estrogen levels decline, so does libido, often leading to a loss of interest in sex or intimacy. This can create tension and conflict in relationships, especially if one partner still desires physical closeness while the other does not. Additionally, factors like vaginal dryness, fatigue, and stress can further dampen sexual desire, exacerbating the situation.

Effective communication and mutual understanding are essential in addressing these challenges. Couples can explore alternative ways of fostering intimacy and connection, such as prioritizing non-sexual affection, scheduling date nights, or seeking medical advice to address physical discomfort. It's essential to approach these conversations with empathy and openness, acknowledging each other's needs and limitations.

- **My mood swings are unbearable for my partner**

Mood swings and irritability can strain even the strongest of relationships. Hormonal fluctuations during

Peri-menopause can lead to heightened emotional sensitivity and difficulty regulating mood, resulting in outbursts of anger or irritability. Partners may struggle to understand why their loved one is behaving this way, often interpreting it as directed towards them.

In such instances, seeking support and exploring coping strategies becomes crucial. Whether through relaxation techniques, lifestyle adjustments, or professional guidance, finding effective ways to manage mood swings can alleviate strain on the relationship.

Additionally, partners can play a supportive role by offering understanding, patience, and encouragement during these challenging times.

While perimenopause can indeed pose challenges to relationships, it also presents an opportunity for growth and deeper connection. By fostering open communication, empathy, and mutual support, couples can navigate the complexities of Peri-menopause together, emerging stronger on the other side. Sharing experiences and seeking guidance can also provide solace and reassurance, reminding us that we're not alone in this journey.

Chapter 5:
Lifestyle Changes for Optimal Wellbeing

Perimenopause is a personal journey, and its impact varies widely from woman to woman. On average, it stretches more than four years. That's a long time to be uncomfortable in your body – to experience the physical and mental symptoms of perimenopause. Beyond these symptoms, women might face other health changes such as cardiometabolic shifts, altered fat distribution, heightened systemic inflammation, and cognitive challenges.

That is why we have to make lifestyle changes that will make this period much more bearable, even fun. Embracing good nutrition, maintaining an active lifestyle, and practicing stress management can significantly enhance well-being during this transition.

The risks of chronic disease and health problems due to declining estrogen levels after menopause are well-documented. However, many studies have grouped peri- and postmenopausal women together, despite their distinct needs and experiences.

Fortunately, recent research is starting to differentiate between these stages, providing clearer insights into managing perimenopause and exploring beneficial lifestyle interventions.

While diet and lifestyle adjustments aren't magic fixes, they can substantially improve your quality of life and might alleviate some of the discomforts associated with perimenopause. Focusing on a balanced diet and healthy habits can prepare you for long-term health and potentially ease some of the common symptoms.

Nutrition and Diet

Aim for a diet rich in fruits, vegetables, whole grains, and low-fat dairy. When perimenopause hits, your body undergoes significant changes and may benefit from additional nutrients.

- **Protein**

During this perimenopause, your body's muscle mass begins to decline. To counteract this, increasing your daily protein intake can be beneficial, according to research.

Protein supports muscle maintenance and helps regulate appetite and blood sugar levels. It might also help in balancing hormones. Spread your protein consumption across meals and snacks—consider topping toast with peanut butter, adding baked salmon or chicken to salads, or including beans in your dinner. Snacks like homemade nut mixes, eggs, lentils, and yogurt are excellent sources of protein.

- **Omega-3 Fatty Acids**

Omega-3 fatty acids are linked to reduced inflammation and improved mood, making them particularly valuable during perimenopause. They may also help alleviate depression, a common issue during this time. Aim for two 4-ounce servings of fish weekly or discuss fish oil supplements with your doctor. Flaxseed oil is another option that might help with mood swings and irritability.

- **Fiber**

Fiber is your friend during perimenopause. It helps you feel fuller for longer, which can help in weight management as your metabolism slows. Additionally, fiber reduces the risk of diseases such as heart disease, stroke, and cancer. Strive for at least 21 grams of fiber daily, found in fruits, vegetables, whole grains, and beans. Avoid overly processed foods, which are typically lower in fiber.

- **Calcium**

With age, the risk of osteoporosis increases. To support bone health, aim for 1,200 milligrams of calcium daily, and don't forget about vitamin D. Consult your doctor for personalized recommendations, as opinions on optimal intake can vary.

Making thoughtful dietary and lifestyle choices can have a profound impact during perimenopause, helping you navigate this transition with greater ease and vitality.

What to Avoid

Navigating the dietary changes that come with perimenopause can feel overwhelming, but some adjustments can make a real difference in how you feel. While no one likes to hear a long list of forbidden foods, it's important to understand which choices might not serve you well. Saturated fats, often found in meat and dairy, are linked to an increased risk of heart disease. Opt for plant-based fats whenever you can for a heart-healthy alternative.

Highly refined carbs—think white breads, pasta, and sugary baked goods—can spike blood sugar levels and lead to persistent cravings. A simple swap, like choosing whole grain brown rice over white rice, can help manage these effects. Additionally, sugar, caffeine, and alcohol can amplify hormone-related symptoms, so cutting back on these can offer some relief.

Note: *If you're a smoker, quitting is one of the best moves for your overall well-being.*

Your body is undergoing significant hormonal shifts during this time, which can bring about many symptoms. Making mindful food choices can help you navigate this transition with greater ease and comfort.

Supplements to Consider

Supporting healthy hormone levels is crucial for managing the symptoms of perimenopause and enhancing your overall well-being. One of the most effective strategies for balancing your hormones is through a diet rich in key nutrients. But sometimes, you are either not getting enough of these nutrients from the food you take, or your body is unable to utilize them well, so that you need supplementation. There are supplements that can bolster your mental and emotional health during perimenopause, backed by research on how they can help counteract the effects of decreasing hormone levels. The idea is to help you live your most vibrant and fulfilling life.

1. Magnesium

Magnesium is crucial for regulating brain function, mood, and stress response. As we age, we tend to consume fewer magnesium-rich foods and our bodies absorb nutrients less efficiently, which can exacerbate chronic stress and lead to deficiencies. A study of 171 postmenopausal women showed that over 80% had low magnesium levels and were more likely to report feelings of depression. Replenishing magnesium can help break this cycle and enhance overall well-being.

Where to naturally get magnesium - Avocado, bananas, pumpkin seeds, spinach, cashews, oatmeal, black beans.

Supplement recommendations - The recommended daily allowance (RDA) for women over 30 is 320 mg, with an upper limit of 350 mg per day.

2. Vitamin D

Often called a vitamin but functioning more like a prohormone, vitamin D helps regulate and protect your dopamine system—key for mood balance. As we age, reduced sun exposure and lower skin production of vitamin D make supplementation and vitamin D-rich foods important.

Where to naturally get vitamin D - Oily fish, egg yolks, milk, plant-based milks, fortified juices, and cereals. Since vitamin D isn't found in fruits and vegetables, it's essential to look for fortified products and enjoy some sun exposure.

How much vitamin D do you need? - The National Institutes of Health recommends 15 mcg (600 IU) per day. Since vitamin D is fat-soluble, excess intake can lead to issues, so consult with your healthcare provider for personalized advice.

3. B Vitamins

B vitamins are essential for energy levels, brain function, and emotional stability. Vitamin B6, folic acid, and B12 are particularly important during perimenopause. B6 helps produce serotonin, which can decline with age and affect mood. Deficiencies in B vitamins can lead to irritability, depression, fatigue, and confusion.

Where to naturally get B vitamins - Tuna, turkey, chicken, salmon, sweet potatoes, nutritional yeast, sunflower seeds, beets, citrus fruits

How much B6, Folic Acid, and B12 do you need?

- Vitamin B6: 1.3 mg (women under 50), 1.5 mg (women 50+)
- Folic Acid: 400 mcg DFE
- Vitamin B12: 2.4 mcg

4. Omega-3 Fatty Acids

Omega-3s are vital for brain health and combating depression. They offer neuroprotective and anti-inflammatory benefits and may help prevent cognitive decline. Studies show that omega-3s can lower the risk of depression and maintain mental health as you age.

Where to naturally get omega-3s - Flaxseeds, walnuts, salmon, beef, chia seeds, soybeans, tofu, Brussels sprouts, cauliflower

How much Omega-3 fatty acids do you need? - For ALA, the recommended intake is 1.1 g per day. The FDA advises no more than 5 g/day of combined EPA and DHA from supplements.

5. Zinc

Zinc supports neurotransmitter synthesis and can alleviate symptoms of depression and anxiety associated with hormonal changes. It also benefits sexual health, which can impact mood and overall mental health.

Where to naturally get zinc - Red meat, oysters, chickpeas, dairy, eggs, hemp seeds, dark chocolate

How much zinc do you need? - The NIH recommends 8 mg per day for women 19+ years old.

6. Probiotics

Probiotics support a healthy gut, which is crucial for mental health since over 95% of serotonin is produced in the gut. Good bacteria in probiotics help stabilize moods, reduce inflammation, and balance hormones, potentially easing symptoms like sleep issues and hot flashes.

Where to naturally get probiotics - Yogurt, kefir, fermented vegetables, kombucha, sauerkraut

How much probiotics should you take? - There are no standardized dosages, so follow the product's label for specific recommendations based on strains and potency.

Regular Exercise

A third of our lives will be spent post-menopause, making it crucial to establish a solid exercise routine starting in perimenopause. Regular physical activity not only enhances quality of life during these years but also helps alleviate perimenopausal symptoms.

Here's why integrating exercise into your daily routine is vital:

- Maintains a healthy weight - Exercise helps in managing weight, which can become more challenging during perimenopause.
- Builds muscle mass - Increased muscle mass protects bones and boosts metabolism, which often slows with age.
- Reduces breast cancer risk - Regular physical activity is linked to a lower risk of breast cancer.

- Decreases stress - Exercise improves general mental well-being and helps manage stress levels.
- Promotes heart health - Regular activity helps in weight management, improves cholesterol levels, and helps prevent type 2 diabetes.
- Improves sleep patterns - Engaging in physical activity can enhance the quality of your sleep.
- Enhances mobility - Regular exercise supports better mobility as you age.

Finding the Right Routine

To make exercise a lasting part of your life, choose activities you enjoy and incorporate them into your daily routine. Exercising with a friend can provide motivation and accountability. Remember to focus on how good you feel after exercising, which can help maintain your commitment.

Even if you already exercise regularly, varying your routine can keep it engaging and effective. Combining cardio and resistance training offers the most benefits.

- Resistance training - This can include weights, but also bodyweight exercises like yoga and Pilates. It's essential for improving muscle mass and bone strength.
- Cardio - Activities like running, cycling, and high-intensity interval training (HIIT) elevate your heart rate, benefiting heart and circulatory health.

Both types of exercise are proven to enhance mental well-being, which you need during perimenopause.

Getting Started

If you're finding it difficult to start, aim for a daily goal of 10,000 steps and build from there. It's always wise to consult with a healthcare professional before beginning a new exercise program, especially if you have health concerns or have been inactive for a while.

You can also incorporate a mix of these activities into your weekly routine to protect and strengthen your heart, bones, and muscles, while also improving balance, mood, and overall well-being:

- Brisk walking
- Jogging
- Biking or spinning
- Aerobics
- Dancing
- Tennis
- Weight training
- Interval training

Regular exercise is crucial for maintaining your health and well-being during and beyond perimenopause. By staying active, you can enjoy a better quality of life. Aim for at least 150 minutes of moderate intensity exercise per week.

Tips for Exercising Well

As we enter our forties and fifties, the approach to fitness must evolve due to physical changes, including slower metabolisms, hormonal shifts, and increased risks of heart and bone issues. Adapting your exercise routine to these changes can significantly impact your health and well-being. Here are some tips to exercise smarter:

1. Follow recommended exercise levels

The World Health Organization and the Centers for Disease Control and Prevention (CDC) recommend adults up to age 64 engage in:

- 150 to 300 minutes of moderate aerobic exercise or
- 75 to 150 minutes of vigorous aerobic exercise per week

This equates to about 30 minutes a day, five to seven days a week. Additionally, it's recommended to incorporate muscle-strengthening activities at least twice a week and to stretch both before and after exercise to prepare the body for optimal performance.

2. Enhance cardiovascular health

With aging, the risk of heart disease increases. To counteract this:

- Engage in 30 minutes of aerobic exercise most days of the week. Activities such as brisk walking, running, biking, or dancing are beneficial.
- Build up your routine gradually to include one high-intensity aerobic session, two to three moderate-intensity sessions, at least one strength training session, and one longer aerobic session each week.

A 2018 study found that participants in their fifties improved heart health by sticking to these exercise guidelines, showing reduced heart stiffness and better overall fitness.

3. Strengthen your bones

Bone density naturally decreases with age, especially due to falling estrogen levels during perimenopause. To combat this:

- Incorporate strength training exercises to build muscle and strengthen bones, which helps prevent falls and fractures. Exercises such as toe-heel raises can be effective:
  - Stand straight, holding onto a chair.
  - Rise onto your toes, then lower back down. Next, tip back on your heels, then lower down.
  - Repeat 10 times, challenging your balance by holding onto the chair as little as possible.
  - Perform this exercise daily.

4. Support mental health and mood

Loneliness and mental health issues often peak in the late fifties. Aerobic exercise has been shown to alleviate anxiety and depression by increasing blood flow and endorphin production. If you're not already getting 30 minutes of cardiovascular exercise most days:

- Try various activities such as jogging, swimming, cycling, walking, gardening, or dancing.
- Aim to gradually build up to 30 minutes a day, which can help improve mood and mental well-being.

5. Integrate interval training

Perimenopause often brings symptoms like hot flashes, irregular periods, and weight gain. While exercise won't eliminate these symptoms, it can help. Incorporate interval training into your routine, alternating between moderate and high-intensity exercises.

For example, walk for five minutes, jog for one minute, then walk again. Repeat the jogging intervals several times.

The North American Menopause Society (NAMS) supports this approach as effective in managing weight and reducing stress.

Note: Whether you're new to exercise or looking to adapt your current routine, remember to:

- *Consult with a healthcare professional before starting a new exercise program, especially if you have health concerns or haven't been active recently.*
- *Mix up your activities to include both cardio and strength training, and alwaysincorporate stretching to prepare and recover your body.*

By adjusting your fitness routine to your changing needs, you can support your heart, bones, and overall health while navigating the transitions of midlife and beyond.

Sleep Hygiene

Sleep disorders are often overlooked in discussions about perimenopause, yet they affect 40-60% of perimenopausal women. These issues are tied to fluctuating estrogen and progesterone levels which disrupt menstrual cycles and sleep patterns. Addressing these disruptions is crucial for maintaining overall well-being.

Recap: Causes of Sleep Problems

1. Hot flashes

Hot flashes are one of the most well-known symptoms of perimenopause and a significant cause of sleep disturbances. They occur when the hypothalamus, the body's temperature regulator, misinterprets your body temperature as being too high. This triggers a cooling response involving hormone release and changes in blood vessel dilation to dissipate excess heat. The result is a sudden feeling of intense warmth, flushing, and sweating, which can be severe enough to soak bed linens and disrupt sleep.

2. Quality of life

Perimenopause often brings physical discomforts that can impact the overall quality of life. Symptoms such as mood swings, weight gain, and vaginal dryness can lead to psychological distress. This distress can make it difficult to relax and fall asleep, exacerbating sleep problems. Additionally, perimenopause coincides with other life changes, such as managing a career, personal responsibilities, and family matters, which can add to the stress and interfere with sleep.

3. Sleep apnea

Sleep apnea is characterized by recurring interruptions in breathing during sleep. It becomes more common in perimenopausal women. This is partly due to hormonal changes that affect muscle tone and fat distribution. A decrease in estrogen and progesterone can relax the throat muscles around the airways, leading to airway obstruction. Perimenopausal women are also more likely to experience weight gain, which can further increase the risk of sleep apnea. This condition can lead to snoring, daytime sleepiness, and an increased risk of cardiovascular problems if left untreated.

Insomnia and perimenopause

Insomnia, defined by difficulty falling or staying asleep, is more prevalent during perimenopause. Several factors contribute to this:

- Hormonal fluctuations - The decline in estrogen and progesterone levels can disrupt serotonin production in the brain. Serotonin is a neurotransmitter that regulates mood and sleep. Changes in these hormone levels can therefore affect sleep patterns, making it harder to fall asleep or stay asleep throughout the night.

- Psychological distress - Peri-menopause often coincides with increased stress and anxiety. Elevated cortisol levels, which rise in response to stress, can spike following a hot flash or other Peri-menopause symptoms. The combination of physical discomforts and the demands of managing various aspects of life can contribute to insomnia. Psychological factors, such as depression or anxiety about aging, can further exacerbate sleep difficulties.

- Diet - Dietary choices can impact sleep quality. Research indicates that a diet high in processed carbohydrates and sugary foods may increase the risk of insomnia. Rapid blood sugar spikes followed by crashes can cause frequent awakenings during the night. In contrast, a diet rich in whole grains, fruits, and vegetables is associated with better sleep outcomes.

Hot Flashes and Night Sweats

The exact cause of hot flashes and night sweats is not fully understood, but they are believed to result from hormonal changes affecting the hypothalamus. This disruption leads to improper temperature regulation, causing the characteristic symptoms.

For some women, hormonal changes are more pronounced at night, leading to more frequent or intense hot flashes during sleep. Besides, at night, you may not be aware of the onset of hot flashes, which can result in sudden awakenings during the most intense episodes.

Not only that, but certain foods and beverages can exacerbate hot flashes. Caffeine, alcohol, spicy foods, and high-GI (glycemic index) foods can increase body temperature and make night sweats worse. Medications taken in the evening may also contribute to these symptoms.

Then, if your environment is not well thought out, it makes it all worse - warm room, heavy blankets, or synthetic bedding can contribute to overheating and worsen night sweats.

We've already established that perimenopausal women are at higher risk for obstructive sleep apnea due to changes in muscle tone and fat distribution. The relaxation of throat muscles and increased neck circumference can lead to airway obstruction. They are also at a higher risk of restless leg syndrome (RLS). RLS is characterized by an uncomfortable sensation in the legs and an uncontrollable urge to move them, often occurring at night. Changes in estrogen levels and low iron levels during Peri-menopause can affect neurotransmitters like dopamine and glutamate, leading to RLS. This condition can interfere with falling asleep and maintaining sleep. RLS is also commonly associated with other disorders like depression and anxiety, which can compound sleep difficulties.

So, then what does good sleep hygiene look like and how can it help you sleep better?

- Create a sleep-friendly environment - Keep your bedroom cool (ideally between 60-67°F or 15.6–19.4°C), dark, and quiet. Removing electronic

devices that emit light can help prevent disruptions in sleep.
- Maintain a regular sleep schedule - Go to bed and wake up at the same time every day to regulate your body's internal clock.
- Establish a bedtime routine - Engage in calming activities before bed, such as reading, taking a warm bath, or listening to soothing sounds. This routine can help signal your body that it's time to wind down.
- Avoid late naps and screen time - Minimize late-day naps and avoid screen exposure before bedtime, as the blue light emitted by screens can interfere with melatonin production, a hormone necessary for sleep.
- Exercise regularly - Regular physical activity can promote better sleep. Activities like brisk walking, gardening, and other moderate exercises can be beneficial. However, avoid vigorous exercise close to bedtime.
- Manage snoring - If snoring is an issue, consider using a mouth guard, adjusting your pillow height, or adding moisture to the air with a humidifier.

Bear in mind that the things you consume also affect your sleep. Limit or avoid alcohol, caffeine, and large meals close to bedtime. These can disrupt sleep patterns and exacerbate menopausal symptoms. It is a good practice to eat your last meal at least 3-4 hours before bedtime. If you need a snack, opt for plant-based options like hummus, fruits, seeds, or nuts. Consider adding sleep friendly supplements to your diet. Herbal supplements like melatonin or valerian root may aid sleep, but consult with your physician before using them to avoid interactions with other medications.

As a thing to note, practices such as yoga, meditation, and aromatherapy can promote relaxation and improve sleep quality. You can also try CBT. CBT for insomnia focuses on changing negative thoughts and behaviors related to sleep. It has been shown to be effective in managing sleep problems. Explore alternative therapies if you need to. Hypnosis and acupuncture may help alleviate Peri-menopause symptoms and improve sleep by redirecting focus away from discomfort.

Stress Management

Many women find perimenopause to be a stressful time. This can be partly due to hormonal changes that bring on symptoms like hot flashes and sleepless nights. On top of that, family issues such as handling teenage kids, adjusting to an empty nest, caring for aging parents, and dealing with career shifts often pile on additional stress.

Stress can affect us in both emotional and physical ways. Emotionally, we might feel overwhelmed or anxious based on how we view and react to situations. Physically, stress can show up as a rapid heartbeat, sweaty palms, or digestive issues. But what does stress have to do with perimenopause?

For some women, perimenopause itself can be a stressor. It's a major life change that can offer a chance to reevaluate aspects of our lives like our careers, relationships, and health. However, fluctuating hormones can make it harder to handle stress, potentially leading to feelings of depression or anxiety. Sometimes, women might not realize these feelings are linked to hormonal changes and might be prescribed antidepressants unnecessarily. Fortunately, there are natural ways to manage these symptoms and reduce stress.

Chronic stress isn't good for anyone's health. It can raise blood pressure, cause headaches, worsen reflux, and increase the risk of heart disease over time. Some believe it may also weaken the immune system, making us more prone to illnesses. Stress affects not only our health but also our relationships, work performance, and overall well-being. So how do you deal with stress?

1. Identify your stress triggers

The first step in managing stress is figuring out what's causing it. Keeping a stress diary can help. When you're stressed, note what happened, how it made you feel, how you reacted, and what helped. Here are some common stress triggers during perimenopause:

- Self-neglect - Skipping meals, staying up late, or self-medicating with alcohol can increase anxiety.
- Processed foods - Foods high in sugar can cause blood sugar spikes and crashes, which can make you feel more anxious.
- Alcohol - Though it might seem to help you unwind, alcohol is a depressant that can actually worsen anxiety.
- Caffeine - Coffee, tea, cola, and energy drinks can make you jittery and anxious. Opt for caffeine-free herbal teas like peppermint or chamomile instead.
- Sleep - Poor sleep is linked to both mental and physical health issues, including anxiety. Improving your sleep hygiene, like reducing screen time before bed and keeping your phone out of the bedroom, can help.

2. Be honest with yourself

Check if you might be contributing to your own stress. For example, if your job is stressing you out, consider if your actions are part of the problem—like being late or procrastinating. If you find that your own habits are adding to your stress, you have the power to change them. If not, you might need to adjust how you respond to the situation or think about finding a new job.

3. Take action

Once you identify your stress triggers, take steps to address them. If running late is causing stress, try getting up earlier or preparing things the night before. Lay out your clothes, make breakfast, and pack your lunch in advance. A little planning can make your mornings smoother and help you start your day less stressed.

By understanding what causes your stress and taking proactive steps, you can better manage your well-being during perimenopause. Incorporate stress management techniques into your daily routine to help you stay calm and balanced. Here are some simple ways to reduce stress:

- Talk it out - Share your concerns with a family member, friend, healthcare professional, or counselor.
- Relax - Try a "mind-body" program if available in your community, or practice deep breathing (like the one provided below), positive thinking, hypnosis, or meditation (example provided below) using books and CDs. Engage in hobbies that help you relax.
- Walking - A simple walk is great for overall well-being and stress management.
- Pamper yourself - Treat yourself to a massage, a manicure, or a relaxing bath. Enjoy a good book, music, or a favorite hobby. Consider joining an art or music class for a creative outlet.

- Journal - Writing down your feelings can be a great way to process them. It can also help you see what needs more attention and how you talk to yourself. Aim to be kind and gentle with yourself.
- Enjoy - Make time to laugh and smile whenever you can.

Breathing technique to try

Deep breathing exercises can help reduce stress. Try this simple technique whenever you feel stressed:

1. Sit up straight with your feet flat on the floor.
2. Place your hands on your abdomen.
3. Inhale slowly through your nose for a count of four, feeling your abdomen rise.
4. Hold your breath for a second.
5. Exhale slowly through your mouth for a count of four, letting your abdomen fall.
6. Repeat 5 to 10 times.

Guided imagery & meditation example

Vacations can be a great stress reliever, but if you can't take one right now, try a mental escape with guided imagery:

1. Close your eyes and visualize a scene from your memory that brings you joy.
2. Immerse yourself in that memory for a few minutes, allowing your mind to relax and enjoy the pleasant experience.

Quick Biology

When you're stressed, your body produces two hormones, cortisol and adrenaline, from the adrenal glands.

These hormones are part of your body's "fight or flight" response, giving you energy and focus but also affecting your health if they are elevated for too long.

During Peri-menopause, your adrenal glands take on some hormone-producing tasks as your ovaries slow down. However, if the adrenals are constantly pumping out stress hormones, they can't produce enough of the essential hormones like estrogen and progesterone. This imbalance can lead to more stress and related symptoms.

Chronic stress can lead to adrenal fatigue, causing symptoms like depression, weight gain, exhaustion, and more. High cortisol levels, which can come from stress, can worsen menopause symptoms, such as:

- Insomnia
- Low energy
- Frequent colds
- Cravings for unhealthy foods
- Digestive issues
- Weight gain, especially around the middle
- Low sex drive
- Aches and pains
- Low mood

Use your perimenopausal years as a time to reflect and address lifestyle factors contributing to your stress. You will notice that other lifestyle changes like exercise and the right nutrition also help with stress relief. Many of the changes you will make are intertwined and their effects cut across the board. As a rule of thumb, though, when it comes to stress and nutrition, maintain balanced blood sugar levels by avoiding foods that cause spikes and crashes. A roller-coaster in blood sugar can lead to more cortisol production.

Mindfulness and Relaxation

Mindfulness and relaxation techniques can be really helpful in handling the emotional and physical changes during perimenopause. Practices like mindfulness meditation, deep breathing, and progressive muscle relaxation can help reduce anxiety, promote emotional balance, and improve overall well-being. You can weave these practices into your daily routine to find a sense of calm and inner peace.

Mindfulness simply means paying full attention to the present moment—being aware of where you are, what you're doing, and how you're feeling. It might sound easy, but we often find our minds drifting away, getting caught up in worries about the past or future, which can increase anxiety.

Being mindful means reconnecting with the here and now, helping you stay grounded and less overwhelmed. While it's hard to fully describe in words, practicing mindfulness regularly can help you experience it firsthand. Even though mindfulness is something we all naturally possess, there are ways to cultivate it:

1. Meditation - Try seated, walking, standing, or even lying down meditation (though lying down can sometimes lead to sleep).
2. Daily pauses - Insert short moments of mindfulness into your everyday life.
3. Combining practices - Integrate mindfulness with other activities, like yoga or sports.

While it's best to focus on the practice rather than the benefits, there are clear advantages to mindfulness including:

- It helps lower stress levels.
- It improves focus and performance in various aspects of life.

- It increases self-awareness and understanding of your own mind.
- It boosts attention to others' well-being.

Mindfulness meditation offers a chance to pause judgment and approach life with curiosity and kindness, both towards yourself and others.

The thing with mindfulness is that it is familiar. It is something we already do in various ways. It's not a new or exotic practice. In fact, I would go as far as say we have the innate ability to be mindful. We all have the ability to be present. Mindfulness helps us tap into this natural skill. Mindfulness doesn't require you to become someone else; it enhances who you already are. It has the power to bring about positive change on a personal and social level.

I also like that mindfulness is accessible to everyone. Anyone can practice mindfulness. It doesn't require changing beliefs and is easy to learn. Anyone can make it into a way of life. Mindfulness isn't just a practice but a way to bring awareness and care into everyday actions, reducing unnecessary stress. And thankfully, its perks are evidence-based. Research shows that mindfulness positively impacts health, happiness, work, and relationships. It can lead to creative and resilient solutions to complex problems.

As you practice mindfulness, you will start to see that it isn't just about thoughts—it's also about being in tune with your body. Meditation starts with awareness of your physical state, which can help you relax and align with your body's natural rhythms. Paying attention to your body's sensations and rhythms can provide a calming effect, grounding you in the present moment.

Mindfulness and relaxation techniques added into your routine are a great way to better manage the changes and challenges of perimenopause, enhancing your overall

well-being and emotional balance. Here's a simple guide to help you get comfortable for meditation, whether you're just starting or taking a moment to center yourself. Feel free to adjust based on your physical needs or any injuries. (More relaxation techniques are provided in the Appendix.)

1. Find your seat - Sit on whatever you're using—be it a chair, cushion, or park bench. Make sure your seat is stable and solid, so you're not perching or leaning back.

2. Check your legs - If you're on a cushion, cross your legs comfortably in front of you. If you're in a chair, make sure your feet are flat on the floor.

3. Straighten up - Sit up straight, but don't stiffen. Your spine naturally curves, so let it do its thing. Your head and shoulders should comfortably align with your spine.

4. Position your arms - Let your upper arms hang naturally at your sides, and place your hands on your thighs. Aim for a position where your hands are neither too far forward (which makes you hunch) nor too far back (which makes you stiff). Find a relaxed, neutral spot.

5. Relax your gaze - Drop your chin slightly and let your gaze fall gently downward. You can lower your eyelids if you like, but it's not essential to close your eyes. Just let your eyes rest naturally without focusing too much on what you see.

6. Take a moment - Sit quietly for a few moments. Relax and focus on your breath or the sensations in your body.

7. Start meditating - Once you're settled, pay attention to your breath. Notice it coming in and going out. If your mind starts to wander, gently bring your focus back to your breath without judging yourself. It's natural for your mind to drift—just return to the breath whenever you notice it.

8. Keep practicing - That's the essence of meditation. It sounds simple, but it can be challenging. The key is to keep practicing regularly. Over time, you'll notice the benefits.

I have found that you can create a comfortable and effective meditation practice that helps you find moments of calm and relaxation in your daily routine. Remember the goal with mindfulness, as with any other lifestyle change discussed in this chapter, the goal is to make it part of your daily habits. Find a balance that works for you and honors your unique experience of perimenopause.

Chapter 6:
Seeking Support and Professional Guidance

Experiencing perimenopause can feel incredibly isolating especially in the initial years. The physical and emotional changes can seem overwhelming, and you might feel like no one truly understands what you're going through. It's common to want to keep these feelings to yourself, but reaching out for support is important.

The stigma around perimenopause and mental health issues can make it hard to open up. You might worry about being judged, which can lead you to hide what you're feeling from coworkers, friends, or even family members.

It's easy to isolate yourself during this time, especially if you're low on energy or unsure of where to seek help. Opening up about perimenopause can be daunting, but it's crucial to find support. Just like with physical health issues, addressing emotional and mental health needs during perimenopause is important. Here's how to recognize when you need support and how to find it:

1. Learn about perimenopause - Understanding perimenopause and its symptoms can help you explain your situation to others, so it is a big win that you are reading this book. People often have misconceptions or limited knowledge about perimenopause, so being able to describe what you're going through can help them understand and

provide better support. By educating yourself, you also educate those around you.

2. Situational awareness - Be aware of external factors that might affect your emotional and mental well-being. Life changes, stress, and health issues can all impact how you feel. Recognizing these factors can help you understand when it's time to seek help. This might not always be easy, as it can be a challenge to acknowledge when you're struggling, especially if you're used to pushing through tough times.

3. Identify supportive people - Find someone you trust who has shown compassion in the past. Look at the support network you built in Chapter 4. This could be a friend, family member, or someone else in your life who you believe will be understanding. Not everyone will know how to support you, so look for those who have proven to be empathetic and caring.

4. Clarify your needs - Before reaching out to someone, think about what you hope to gain from the conversation. Are you looking for someone to listen, or do you need practical help with tasks? Being specific about your needs can help the person understand how best to support you. For example, you might say, "I'm feeling overwhelmed and need someone to talk to," or "I'm struggling with daily tasks and could use some help."

5. Maintain your support network - Try to create a network of people you can turn to for support. Relying on just one person can be risky, as they might not always be available. Having a group of supportive friends and family ensures that you

have multiple sources of help when you need it. Remember to give back in these relationships as well so that they are reciprocal.

If you find it challenging to locate support within your immediate circle, remember that there are other resources available. Therapists, support groups, and community organizations can offer valuable assistance. Even if your family and friends are limited, professionals and volunteers can provide the support you need.

By reaching out and expressing your needs, you not only help yourself but also contribute to breaking down the stigma surrounding perimenopause. Each time you share your experience, you make it easier for others to do the same, creating a more supportive environment for everyone.

Healthcare Professional Guidance

Navigating perimenopause can be challenging, and consulting with a healthcare professional is essential during this transition. Here's why:

1. Personalized guidance - Every woman's experience with perimenopause is unique. A healthcare professional can offer tailored advice based on your specific symptoms and needs. Whether you're dealing with hot flashes, mood swings, or sleep disturbances, they can help you understand what's happening in your body and suggest appropriate strategies to manage these changes.

2. Answering your questions - Perimenopause often brings up many questions and concerns. From hormone therapy options to lifestyle changes, having a healthcare professional to discuss these topics can provide clarity and reassurance. They can

explain what to expect during this phase and help you make informed decisions about your health.

3. Regular check-ups - Regular check-ups are crucial during perimenopause to monitor your overall health. Your healthcare provider will keep track of important health indicators like bone density, cholesterol levels, and breast health. This proactive approach helps catch any potential issues early and ensures that you're on top of your health during this transitional period.

4. Screenings and preventative care - Perimenopause can affect various aspects of your health, so regular screenings are essential. For instance, bone density tests can help assess your risk for osteoporosis, while cholesterol checks are important for cardiovascular health. Breast exams and mammograms are also crucial to ensure your breast health remains stable.

5. Managing symptoms - A healthcare professional can recommend treatments or therapies to alleviate perimenopausal symptoms. Whether it's hormonal treatments, lifestyle adjustments, or alternative therapies, they can help you find what works best for you. Their expertise ensures that your treatment plan is safe and effective.

Consulting with a healthcare professional during perimenopause provides you with essential support and guidance. They help you manage symptoms, monitor your health, and make informed decisions about your care. Regular check-ups and screenings are vital to maintaining your overall well-being as you navigate this significant life transition.

What to Expect for Each Test

1. Bone Density

A bone density test, or DEXA scan, is a straightforward and painless procedure that measures the strength of your bones. Here's what you can expect:

Preparing for the Test

You don't need to do anything special to prepare for the scan.

You may be able to keep your clothes on, but you'll need to remove any items with metal fasteners, like zippers or hooks. In some cases, you might be asked to wear a hospital gown.

During the Scan

Positioning - You'll lie on your back on a flat X-ray table. It's important to stay still to ensure clear images.

Scanning process - A radiographer, a specialist who performs X-rays, will operate the scanner. A large arm will move over your body, sending a narrow beam of low-dose rays through the area being examined. This is usually your hip and lower spine, but sometimes other parts like the forearm may be scanned depending on your condition and the quality of the scan at the hip or spine.

How it works - The X-rays pass through your body, with some absorbed by tissues like fat and bone. An X-ray detector measures how many X-rays have passed through, and this information is used to create an image of your bone density.

Duration and After the Test

The scan typically takes about 10 to 20 minutes. Once it's done, you can go home right away.

Understanding Your Results

Your bone density is compared to what is expected for a healthy young adult and for someone of your own age, gender, and ethnicity. You will see results for your T Score and Z Score.

- T Score - Measures how your bone density compares to that of a young healthy adult. Scores are classified as follows:
  - Above -1 SD: Normal
  - Between -1 and -2.5 SD: Mildly reduced bone density
  - At or below -2.5 SD: Osteoporosis
- Z Score - Measures how your bone density compares to others of your same age. A Z score below -2 indicates lower than expected bone density for your age.

While the scan provides a good indication of bone strength, it doesn't predict if you will have a fracture. Other factors like age, sex, and past falls also affect fracture risk. Your doctor will use your results along with other risk factors to decide if treatment is needed.

2. Cholesterol Levels

A cholesterol test is a simple and important way to monitor your heart health, especially during perimenopause when your risk factors can change. Here's a guide to what you can expect:

Before the Test

Fasting or non-fasting - Your doctor will let you know if you need to fast before the test. Fasting means not eating or drinking anything except water for 9 to 12 hours before the test. If you don't fast, the test might only provide information about your total cholesterol and HDL (good) cholesterol levels.

You might be asked to remove any clothing with metal fasteners, but generally, you can keep your clothes on. Sometimes, a hospital gown may be provided.

During the Test

Sample collection - A healthcare professional will draw a small sample of your blood, usually from a vein in your arm. The procedure is quick and generally causes minimal discomfort. If more tests are needed, all blood samples are typically taken at the same time.

The blood sample is sent to a laboratory where levels of different types of cholesterol (HDL and LDL) and triglycerides are measured. If you didn't fast, the results might be limited to total cholesterol and HDL cholesterol.

After the Test

The results will show your cholesterol levels in milligrams per deciliter of blood (mg/dL). Your doctor will interpret these results in the context of your age, sex, family history, and other risk factors like smoking, diabetes, and high blood pressure.

Understanding Your Results

- Cholesterol types:

- Total cholesterol - The sum of all cholesterol in your blood.
- LDL cholesterol - Often called "bad cholesterol" because high levels can clog arteries.
- HDL cholesterol - Known as "good cholesterol" as it helps clear LDL from the arteries.
- Triglycerides - A type of fat in the blood that can increase heart disease risk if elevated.

Your cholesterol levels will be compared to healthy ranges:

- Total cholesterol - Below 200 mg/dL is desirable
- LDL cholesterol - Below 100 mg/dL is ideal
- HDL cholesterol - At or above 60 mg/dL is good
- Triglycerides - Below 150 mg/dL is preferred

Frequency of Testing

The American Heart Association suggests checking cholesterol levels every 4 to 6 years for adults starting at age 20, provided there are no high-risk factors. After age 40, your doctor may calculate your 10-year risk for heart disease or stroke and may recommend more frequent testing if needed.

People with cardiovascular disease or other risk factors may need more regular checks.

Additional Considerations

Screening locations - Your primary care doctor is the best person to conduct and interpret your cholesterol test due to their understanding of your overall health. Public screenings may provide basic cholesterol information but might not be as comprehensive.

If you have cholesterol tests done elsewhere, make sure to share these results with your primary care doctor to ensure a complete assessment of your cardiovascular risk.

Getting regular cholesterol tests is a key part of maintaining heart health, especially as you navigate perimenopause and potential changes in your risk factors.

3. Breast Screening

Breast screening, or a mammogram, is a routine procedure to check for any signs of breast issues. Here's what you can expect during the screening process:

Before your appointment

The entire appointment will take about 30 minutes, though the actual mammograms only take a few minutes.

Upon arrival, the mammographer will review your details and ask if you've experienced any breast problems recently. They will also explain the procedure and answer any questions you might have.

During the screening

You'll need to undress from the waist up in a private changing area. You might be given a hospital gown to wear.

- The Procedure
    1. Initial setup - You'll be called into the X-ray room where the mammographer will explain the process.
    2. First mammogram - Your breast will be placed on the X-ray machine and compressed between two plastic plates to keep it still. This only takes

a few seconds, and it's important to stay still during the X-ray.
3. Side view - The machine will be adjusted to capture another angle of your breast, and the process will be repeated.
4. The same procedure will be done for your other breast.

After both mammograms are completed, you'll return to the changing area to get dressed.

In most cases, your results will be mailed to you. It might take some time to receive them, so be patient.

Important Information

Mammograms can be uncomfortable or even painful for some people. The mammographer is trained to support you through the process and help you feel as comfortable as possible. You can ask them to stop at any time if you need to.

Don't use talcum powder or spray deodorants on the day of your appointment, as they can affect the results. Roll-on deodorants are fine. Opt for a skirt or trousers instead of a dress to make undressing easier. Take off any necklaces and nipple piercings before your appointment. Inform the staff if you've had discomfort during past screenings, or if you feel nervous or embarrassed. They are there to help and can use language that makes you feel more at ease.

Note: Any discomfort from the mammogram should subside quickly. If you experience significant pain that persists for more than a couple of days, contact your GP.

Breast screening is a vital part of monitoring your breast health, especially during perimenopause, and understanding what to expect can help make the process smoother and less stressful.

Questions to Ask Your Healthcare Provider

When discussing perimenopause with your healthcare provider, it's helpful to keep a record of your menstrual cycles, noting when they start and end, and how heavy they are. This can give your provider a clearer picture of what you're experiencing. Here are some important questions to ask:

- Are these symptoms related to perimenopause?
- What can I do to manage or ease these symptoms?
- How long might these symptoms last?
- Would hormone therapy be a good option for me?
- Do I need to start any new medications or vitamins?
- Are there any tests I should have?

Always, if your perimenopausal symptoms are severe or affecting your daily life, it's time to reach out to your healthcare provider. They can suggest treatments to help lessen your symptoms and improve your well-being.

Mental Health Support

Navigating the emotional landscape during perimenopause can be challenging. The physical and hormonal changes that occur during this period can impact your mental health significantly. Seeking mental health support can be a vital step in managing these changes effectively. Here's what you need to know about seeking help and what to expect:

When to Seek Help

It's crucial to recognize when you might need professional support. If you're experiencing significant emotional difficulties or mental health challenges during perimenopause, don't hesitate to reach out for help. It's common to feel uncertain about whether your feelings warrant professional support, but it's always okay to seek assistance. Consider seeking help if you:

- Are feeling more anxious or worried than usual
- Struggle to find joy or satisfaction in your daily life
- Experience thoughts or feelings that are overwhelming and affecting your daily functioning
- Want to explore additional support or treatment options

Recap - Emotional Challenges Of Perimenopause

Perimenopause can bring a range of emotional and psychological changes. These challenges may include:

- Hormonal fluctuations - Decreases in estrogen and progesterone can contribute to mood swings, anxiety, and depression. Physical symptoms like hot flashes and night sweats can add to your stress and discomfort.
- Life transitions - This phase often involves significant life changes, such as dealing with aging, possible loss of family members, or children leaving home. These transitions can exacerbate feelings of stress and uncertainty.
- Social isolation - If you feel that friends and family do not fully understand what you're going through, it can lead to feelings of isolation and frustration. This lack of support may also heighten feelings of anxiety or depression.

While everyone experiences periods of sadness, persistent feelings of sadness, hopelessness, or emptiness may signal depression. Key symptoms include:

- Persistent irritability, frustration, or anger
- Increased anxiety, restlessness, or agitation
- Feelings of guilt or worthlessness
- Loss of interest in activities you once enjoyed
- Difficulty concentrating or making decisions
- Memory issues
- Chronic fatigue or lack of energy
- Changes in sleep patterns (either too much or too little)
- Altered appetite or weight changes
- Unexplained physical aches and pains

Several factors can increase the risk of developing depression during perimenopause, including: a history of depression prior to menopause, negative feelings about aging or perimenopause itself, high levels of stress from work, personal relationships, or financial issues, low self-esteem or chronic anxiety, feeling unsupported by those around you, lack of physical activity or exercise, smoking or other unhealthy habits.

Getting the Right Support

Depression during perimenopause is treatable. It's essential to talk to your healthcare provider about the symptoms you're experiencing. They can guide you to the most effective treatment options, which may include:

- Therapy - A mental health professional, such as a therapist or counselor, can provide a safe space to explore your feelings, offer coping strategies, and support your emotional well-being.

- Medication - In some cases, medication may be prescribed to help manage symptoms of depression or anxiety.
- Lifestyle changes - Incorporating regular exercise, a healthy diet, and stress management techniques can also be beneficial.

Taking the step to seek help is a sign of strength, not weakness. By addressing your mental health needs during perimenopause, you can improve your overall well-being and navigate this transition more smoothly.

Support Groups and Online Communities

Connecting with other women who are undergoing similar challenges can provide a crucial support system and valuable resources during perimenopause. There are a number of benefits to joining support groups and online communities:

1. A sense of camaraderie

Support groups and online communities offer a unique space for women experiencing perimenopause to come together and share their journeys. The feeling of camaraderie that arises from these interactions can be incredibly comforting. Knowing that others are facing the same struggles can reduce feelings of isolation and loneliness, and help you realize that you are not alone in this journey.

- Emotional support - Engaging with others who understand your experiences can provide emotional relief and validation. It's reassuring to know that others have similar symptoms and are managing them, which can help you feel more supported and less overwhelmed.

- Shared experiences - Many women find comfort in hearing how others are coping with perimenopause. Whether it's managing hot flashes, dealing with mood swings, or navigating changes in libido, sharing personal stories can offer practical advice and emotional solidarity.

2. Valuable insights and advice

Support groups and online forums can be a treasure trove of information, offering practical tips and advice from those who have been through or are currently navigating perimenopause. This collective wisdom can be incredibly valuable. Members often share effective strategies for dealing with common symptoms. These might include dietary changes, exercise routines, or natural remedies that have worked for others.

You might also receive recommendations for healthcare providers, treatments, or therapies that others have found beneficial. This can help you make more informed decisions about your own care.

3. Empowerment through shared knowledge

Participating in support groups and online communities can be empowering. Sharing knowledge and experiences with others can boost your confidence and help you feel more in control of your health and well-being.

These support groups provide access to a wide range of experiences and opinions that can help you make more informed decisions about your treatment and lifestyle.

Understanding what has worked for others can guide you in finding what might work best for you.

Additionally, being part of a community can increase your awareness of perimenopause and its effects. This can lead to better self-care practices and more proactive management of symptoms. Support from peers can provide motivation to take positive steps towards managing your health. Celebrating small victories and milestones with others can boost your morale and commitment to your health goals.

4. Emotional comfort and understanding

The emotional support provided by these groups can be profound. Perimenopause can bring about significant changes and challenges, and having a space where you can express your feelings and receive understanding can be incredibly comforting:

It's normal to experience a range of emotions during perimenopause. Connecting with others who understand what you're going through can validate your feelings and help you process them in a supportive environment.

Having conversations with people who empathize with your struggles can also reduce stress and anxiety. Sharing your concerns and hearing others' perspectives can help you feel more grounded and less alone.

How to Find Support Groups and Online Communities

There are various ways to find support groups and online communities dedicated to perimenopause:

- Local support groups - Check with local health organizations, community centers, or women's health clinics to find in-person support groups.
- Online forums and social media - Many online platforms host forums and social media groups

focused on perimenopause. Websites like Reddit, Facebook, and specialized health forums offer spaces to connect with others.

- Healthcare providers - Ask your healthcare provider for recommendations on support groups or online communities that they trust.

Engaging with support groups and online communities, can give you comfort, valuable insights, and connection with others who are navigating the challenges of perimenopause.

Chapter 7:
Hormonal and Non-Hormonal Treatment Options

As I've explored various ways to manage the symptoms, I've found that blending conventional treatments with alternative therapies has been particularly effective. This chapter delves into the dual approach of Hormone Replacement Therapy (HRT) and alternative remedies, drawing from both modern medicine and time-tested natural solutions.

One significant aspect of my personal strategy has been embracing herbal remedies, a practice I've adopted with the invaluable help of my Jamaican mum. She is a wealth of knowledge when it comes to natural healing, and her dedication to preparing these remedies has greatly benefited me throughout my perimenopausal journey.

Herbal treatments have been instrumental in alleviating some of the more challenging symptoms I've encountered. For instance, hot flushes, which can be both uncomfortable and disruptive, have been eased by certain herbal concoctions. Similarly, herbal remedies have provided relief from vaginal dryness and supported bone health, particularly for my knees, which have been a concern during this time.

It's worth noting that some of these herbal remedies have a notably bitter taste, a characteristic that my mum insists is a mark of their potency. Her wisdom has taught me that what may be unpleasant to the palate often holds the greatest benefits for the body. This perspective has encouraged me to persist with these remedies, understanding that their efficacy outweighs the initial discomfort of their flavor.

In this chapter, we'll explore how Hormone Replacement Therapy and these alternative herbal approaches can complement each other, offering a holistic approach to managing perimenopause. By blending the benefits of modern medicine with the traditional wisdom of herbal remedies, you can tailor a treatment plan that addresses both physical and emotional aspects of this transitional phase.

Understanding HRT

Hormone replacement therapy (HRT) involves taking medication that provides female hormones to replace the estrogen your body no longer produces during perimenopause. This treatment is primarily aimed at easing common menopausal symptoms such as hot flashes and vaginal dryness.

Additionally, HRT has been found to help prevent bone loss and reduce the risk of fractures in postmenopausal women.

It's important to note that while the terms "hormone therapy" and "hormone replacement therapy" are often used interchangeably, they can have different connotations. Hormone therapy (HT) is a broader term that encompasses any treatment involving hormones, including those used for conditions like cancer or various hormonal imbalances. When referring specifically to menopausal and perimenopausal treatment, the term "hormone replacement therapy" is more commonly used.

Your healthcare provider might choose the term based on your age and context. Generally, "hormone replacement therapy" is used when discussing treatments aimed at replacing hormones that are no longer being produced, especially in individuals in their 30s or early 40s. It's crucial to understand that the risks associated with HRT can vary depending on your age and individual health profile. HRT should be personalized and regularly reviewed to ensure that its benefits outweigh any potential risks.

Purpose of HRT

- Relieving common symptoms - Hormone Replacement Therapy (HRT) is designed to alleviate the common symptoms of menopause, such as hot flashes, night sweats, vaginal dryness, and mood swings. By supplementing the hormones that your body no longer produces in adequate amounts, HRT can significantly reduce the intensity and frequency of these symptoms.

- Preventing bone loss - Estrogen is crucial for maintaining bone density. During menopause, reduced estrogen levels can lead to osteoporosis. HRT helps mitigate this risk by providing estrogen, which supports bone health and reduces the likelihood of fractures.

- Managing urogenital symptoms - Menopause can affect the urogenital system, leading to symptoms like vaginal dryness, urinary urgency, and sexual discomfort. HRT can address these issues by improving moisture and comfort in the vaginal area, as well as alleviating urinary symptoms.

Types of HRT

1. Estrogen therapy - This involves taking estrogen alone and is generally prescribed for women who have had a hysterectomy. Estrogen therapy is available in several forms:
   - Oral tablets - Taken daily, these are the most common form of HRT.
   - Patches - Adhere to the skin and release estrogen over time.
   - Topical gels or creams - Applied directly to the skin, allowing the hormone to be absorbed.
   - Vaginal rings or creams - Inserted into the vagina or applied around it to target local symptoms.
2. Combination therapy - This type of HRT combines estrogen with progesterone (or progestin, a synthetic form of progesterone). It is used for women who still have a uterus to prevent the risk of uterine cancer, which can be heightened by estrogen alone. Forms include:
   - Oral pills - Contain both estrogen and progesterone.
   - Skin patches - Deliver a steady dose of both hormones.
   - Intrauterine devices (IUDs) - Inserted into the uterus to provide localized hormone delivery.

Delivery Methods

1. Oral tablets

These are the most common methods of HRT, taken by mouth on a daily basis. They provide a systemic approach, affecting the whole body.

One significant advantage of oral tablets is their convenience; they are easy to use and require just a single daily dose. They are also well-established and supported by a broad base of research. However, oral tablets can have some downsides. They may increase the risk of blood clots and impact liver function due to the way they are metabolized through the digestive system. Some women may experience gastrointestinal side effects, such as nausea or indigestion.

2. Transdermal patches

Applied to the skin, these patches release hormones gradually into the bloodstream. They offer a continuous delivery of hormones without the need for daily dosing.

The primary benefit of transdermal patches is that they avoid the gastrointestinal tract, potentially reducing the risk of liver-related side effects and gastrointestinal discomfort. Patches also offer convenience, requiring only a weekly or biweekly change, depending on the product. On the downside, some users might experience skin irritation or allergic reactions at the patch site. Sometimes, ensuring that the patch adheres properly and stays in place can sometimes be challenging.

3. Topical creams or gels

Applied directly to the skin, these formulations allow for hormone absorption through the skin. They are suitable for those who prefer not to take oral medication.

One of the advantages of topical HRT is that it allows for localized application, which can be particularly beneficial for addressing specific symptoms like skin dryness or irritation. What's more, this method avoids the gastrointestinal tract, which can be beneficial for those who experience digestive side effects from oral tablets. Even so, topical creams and gels require consistent application and proper dosing, which might be less convenient compared to other methods. There is also a potential risk of transferring the hormones to others through skin contact, which necessitates careful handling and application.

4. Vaginal preparations

Specifically designed for addressing vaginal symptoms, these include creams, rings, and tablets that are applied or inserted into the vaginal area to improve local symptoms such as dryness and discomfort.

One significant advantage is their ability to directly treat symptoms without affecting the entire body, which can reduce systemic side effects. Vaginal preparations are particularly effective for localized symptoms and can be very helpful for women experiencing significant vaginal dryness or irritation. But these products are not suitable for addressing systemic symptoms like hot flashes or night sweats. Understandably, some women may find the application or insertion of these preparations uncomfortable or inconvenient.

How HRT Works

HRT aims to compensate for the decline in estrogen and progesterone production during perimenopause. By replenishing these hormones, HRT helps to alleviate its symptoms and support overall health. It is important to discuss with your healthcare provider the potential benefits and risks associated with HRT, as individual responses and risks may vary.

How Often to Take HRT

HRT is often prescribed at the lowest effective dose and for the shortest duration necessary to manage symptoms.

- Estrogen-only therapy - Typically administered daily. The specific form of estrogen (pill, patch, gel, etc.) and dosage will be determined by your healthcare provider based on your needs.
- Combination therapy
  - ❖ Continuous-combined therapy - Involves taking both estrogen and progesterone daily, in whatever form is prescribed.
  - ❖ Cyclic therapy (Sequential therapy) - Involves taking estrogen every day, with progesterone taken for 12 to 15 days each month.

    Progesterone is commonly administered in pill form during the cycling phase.

Your healthcare provider will work with you to develop a personalized HRT plan that aligns with your symptoms, health history, and preferences. Regular follow-ups are essential to monitor the effectiveness of the therapy and make any necessary adjustments.

Risks and Considerations

Hormone Replacement Therapy (HRT) can offer significant benefits for managing perimenopausal symptoms, but it also carries potential risks that should be carefully considered. Research suggests that for many women, the advantages of HRT may outweigh the risks. However, it's essential to be aware of the potential adverse effects:

1. Endometrial cancer - Women who take estrogen without progestin and still have their uterus may face an increased risk of endometrial cancer.
2. Blood clots - There is a risk of developing blood clots, which can lead to serious complications.
3. Stroke - HRT may elevate the risk of stroke.
4. Breast cancer - The use of HRT can be associated with a heightened risk of breast cancer.

To potentially mitigate these risks, consider the following strategies:

- Timing - Starting HRT within 10 years of menopause (during perimenopause) or before the age of 60 may reduce some of the associated risks.
- Dosage - Using the lowest effective dose for the shortest duration necessary can help manage risks.
- Progestin use - If you have not had a hysterectomy, incorporating progesterone or progestin can lower the risk of endometrial cancer.
- Alternative forms - Exploring different methods of HRT such as patches, gels, mists, vaginal creams, suppositories, or rings might be beneficial.
- Monitoring - Regular mammograms and pelvic exams are important to track any changes and manage risks effectively.

Who Should Avoid HRT?

Certain medical conditions might make HRT less suitable. If you have any of the following conditions, it may be advisable to avoid HRT:

- A history or risk of blood clots can complicate HRT use.
- If you have or have had cancer, such as breast, uterine, or ovarian cancer, HRT might not be appropriate.
- Heart, liver, or gallbladder disease - These conditions can be exacerbated by HRT.
- Heart attack or stroke - A history of heart attack or stroke could increase risks associated with HRT.
- Known or suspected pregnancy is a contraindication for HRT.
- Unexplained vaginal bleeding - This requires evaluation before starting HRT.

If you smoke, your healthcare provider may recommend quitting before initiating HRT, as smoking can increase the risk of complications.

Potential Side Effects

HRT can come with side effects. If you experience any of the following, consult your doctor:

- Bloating
- Breast Swelling or Tenderness
- Headaches
- Mood Changes
- Nausea
- Vaginal Bleeding

Determining If HRT Is Right for You

Deciding whether HRT is appropriate involves evaluating the benefits in relation to your individual health profile. To help guide this decision, consider discussing the following questions with your doctor:

- Are there specific reasons based on my medical history that would make HRT unsuitable for me?
- Could HRT alleviate my symptoms, particularly hot flashes, sleep disturbances related to night sweats, or vasomotor symptoms?
- What alternatives might be effective for managing vaginal dryness, such as vaginal moisturizers?
- Given my past experiences with hormonal treatments, such as birth control pills, should I be concerned about potential side effects?
- How does my family medical history affect my suitability for HRT? For instance, could it help reduce my risk of osteoporosis if it runs in the family, or should concerns about a family history of breast cancer be considered?
- What type of HRT is likely to be most effective for my symptoms and health needs?

Your healthcare provider can help you weigh these considerations and tailor a treatment plan that aligns with your health goals and risks.

Alternative Therapies

Herbal treatments are increasingly explored as alternative or complementary options for managing the symptoms of perimenopause. Although scientific research on many herbal remedies is limited and their effectiveness can vary, certain herbs have been traditionally used for symptom relief and may offer benefits for some women.

1. Black Cohosh

This is one of the most well-known herbs used to alleviate menopausal symptoms, particularly hot flashes and night sweats. It is thought to have estrogen-like effects that can help balance hormones. Some studies suggest it may be effective, but results are mixed, and it is important to use it under the guidance of a healthcare provider.

Black cohosh has been used for over two centuries as a remedy for perimenopausal symptoms, including hot flashes, mood swings, and sleep disturbances. Historically, Native Americans first recognized its benefits, and its use has since spread to Europe, where it has been approved for managing perimenopausal symptoms for more than 40 years.

Research supports the effectiveness of black cohosh in alleviating some menopausal symptoms. Early studies in Germany highlighted its benefits in reducing physical and psychological symptoms such as hot flashes, night sweats, and vaginal dryness. Notably, a study involving 120 women demonstrated that black cohosh was more effective than the antidepressant fluoxetine (Prozac) in reducing hot flashes and night sweats.

Despite its benefits, the efficacy and safety of black cohosh remain subjects of debate. While a 2010 review indicated that it could reduce hot flashes and night sweats by 26%, and more recent studies have linked it to reduced sleep disturbances, not all research supports these findings. The American College of Obstetricians and Gynecologists (ACOG) has pointed out that many early studies were not well-designed and did not assess long-term safety beyond six months. A 2009 study, for instance, found no significant difference in hot flash relief between black cohosh and a placebo. As a result, some experts advise limiting its use to less than six months.

In addition to its use for perimenopausal symptoms, black cohosh has been explored for its potential benefits in other areas. Preliminary studies suggest it may help alleviate premenstrual syndrome (PMS) and menstrual pain.

In terms of preparation, black cohosh is available in various forms, including capsules, tablets, tinctures, and extracts. *The recommended dose ranges from 20 to 80 mg per day, with standardized preparations often preferred for consistency.* Teas made from dried roots are less effective compared to standardized extracts.

As with any herbal treatment, black cohosh should be used with caution. Potential side effects include abdominal pain, dizziness, and nausea, and it may interact with other medications or conditions. Women with hormone-sensitive conditions, liver issues, or those who are pregnant or breastfeeding should avoid black cohosh.

2. Red Clover

Red clover (Trifolium pratense) has long been used as a herbal remedy, particularly for managing symptoms associated with perimenopause. This plant contains phytoestrogens, which are plant-based compounds that mimic the effects of estrogen in the body. It is commonly employed to help alleviate hot flashes and improve bone health. Despite its traditional use and some supportive research, further studies are needed to confirm its efficacy and safety.

Red clover is a wild perennial herb that belongs to the legume family. Historically, it has been utilized for various medicinal purposes, including the treatment of respiratory issues, skin conditions, and menstrual discomfort. Its therapeutic properties are largely attributed to its content of isoflavones, which have estrogen-like effects.

The isoflavones found in red clover are thought to help mitigate symptoms such as hot flashes and night sweats due to their estrogen-mimicking properties. Some studies have suggested that red clover may significantly reduce these symptoms. For instance, certain proprietary extracts of red clover isoflavones have shown promise in managing hot flashes. However, the results are not uniformly positive; the largest studies have sometimes found no significant benefit.

Red clover is available in various forms, including teas, tinctures, capsules, and standardized extracts. The dosage can vary depending on the form used. Generally, *for dried herbs used in tea, 1 to 2 teaspoons of dried flowers steeped in 8 ounces of hot water, consumed 2 to 3 times daily*, is recommended. *For powdered herbs in capsules, typical doses range from 40 to 160 mg per day*. Tinctures and fluid extracts are also options, with specific dosing instructions depending on the concentration.

While red clover is often well-tolerated, it is important to approach its use with caution. Some common side effects reported include headaches, nausea, and rash. Concerns have been raised about its potential to increase bleeding risk, especially when combined with blood-thinning medications. Women with a history of breast cancer or those currently receiving treatment should consult a healthcare provider before using red clover, as it may interact with estrogen-related therapies and tamoxifen.

Because red clover can influence the metabolism of certain medications processed by the liver, it is crucial to discuss its use with a healthcare professional if you are on other medications.

3. Dong Quai

Dong Quai, a well-known herb in traditional Chinese medicine, is often used to manage various menstrual and perimenopausal symptoms. This herb, also called Angelica sinensis, is valued for its potential to support hormonal balance and overall menstrual health. However, its effectiveness specifically for perimenopausal symptoms is not fully established, and caution is advised due to potential interactions with other medications.

Dong Quai has been used for over 2,000 years, primarily for its supposed benefits in "enriching" the blood and improving circulation. It is frequently referred to as the "female ginseng" due to its traditional use in addressing menstrual issues, such as cramps and irregular cycles, as well as menopausal symptoms like hot flashes.

The herb contains various active compounds, including ligustilide, which is believed to have antispasmodic effects that may help alleviate menstrual cramps. Despite this, scientific evidence supporting Dong Quai's effectiveness for perimenopause remains inconclusive. Some studies suggest it might reduce hot flashes, but others have found no significant benefit compared to placebo.

Dong Quai is available in multiple forms, such as teas, capsules, tinctures, and extracts. For managing menstrual symptoms, it is commonly prepared as a tea from dried root or taken in standardized capsule form. Typical dosages can vary, but general recommendations include consuming *1 to 2 teaspoons of dried root steeped in hot water for tea, or 40 to 160 mg of powdered herb in capsules daily.*

Potential side effects include headaches, nausea, and increased bleeding risk. Due to its estrogen-like effects, it may not be suitable for women with hormone-sensitive conditions like breast cancer. Interactions with medications are also a concern. Dong Quai can potentially affect the metabolism of drugs processed by the liver and may interact with blood thinners, hormonal therapies, and other medications. Therefore, it is crucial to consult with a healthcare provider before starting Dong Quai to ensure it is appropriate for your situation and to avoid adverse interactions.

4. Evening Primrose Oil

Evening primrose oil, derived from the seeds of the evening primrose plant (Oenothera biennis), is a popular herbal remedy for managing perimenopause symptoms. It contains gamma-linolenic acid (GLA), an omega-6 fatty acid thought to influence hormone-like substances called prostaglandins, which may help alleviate certain perimenopausal symptoms.

Many women use evening primrose oil to address issues such as mood swings, hot flashes, breast tenderness, and insomnia. However, while anecdotal reports suggest benefits, scientific evidence supporting its effectiveness for these symptoms is limited and mixed. Proponents believe that by boosting prostaglandin levels, the oil may help counterbalance hormonal fluctuations associated with menopause.

Despite its popularity, research on evening primrose oil for menopausal symptoms has not consistently shown strong results. For instance, a 2015 survey published in *Menopause* found that while evening primrose oil is commonly used among postmenopausal women, its efficacy remains under debate. Similarly, a review in *American Family Physician* in 2009 concluded that there is insufficient evidence to confirm its benefits for most clinical indications, including menopause-related symptoms.

In a 2013 study published in *Archives of Gynecology and Obstetrics*, women taking evening primrose oil reported some improvement in the severity of hot flashes, but no significant change in their frequency or duration. This indicates that while some women may experience relief, results can vary.

Evening primrose oil is generally considered safe for most people, though side effects can occur. Common issues include upset stomach, headache, nausea, and diarrhea.

More serious but rare side effects might include increased bruising or bleeding, low blood sugar, allergic reactions, or seizures. It is advised to avoid evening primrose oil if you have bleeding disorders, epilepsy, or are taking certain medications like blood thinners, specific antidepressants, or medications for schizophrenia. It should also be discontinued at least two weeks before any scheduled surgery.

Before starting evening primrose oil, it is important to consult with a healthcare provider to ensure it is suitable for your individual needs and to discuss any potential interactions with medications or other health conditions.

5. Chaste Tree Berry (Vitex)

Chaste Tree Berry, also known as Vitex, is a traditional herbal remedy used to manage various symptoms associated with perimenopause. Derived from the dried fruit of the chaste tree (Vitex agnus-castus), this herb is believed to influence hormone levels and help alleviate issues such as mood swings, hot flashes, and irritability. Some women report benefits, but its overall effectiveness and safety for managing perimenopause symptoms warrant further research.

Historically, Chaste Tree Berry has been utilized for its potential effects on the pituitary gland, which plays a crucial role in regulating hormone production. This herb is thought to help stabilize hormonal fluctuations by influencing the pituitary's function, thereby promoting a balance in estrogen and progesterone levels. This adaptogenic action—where the herb supports the body in either enhancing hormonal deficiencies or calming excesses—may contribute to its effects on perimenopause symptoms.

Chaste Tree Berry is believed to work by modulating the pituitary gland's release of follicle-stimulating hormone (FSH) and luteinizing hormone (LH), which are integral to regulating the menstrual cycle. By stabilizing these hormones, Chaste Tree Berry may help ease the symptoms associated with perimenopause. Some studies suggest that it may help reduce hot flashes, night sweats, and mood disturbances. For instance, a 2011 study found that women taking Chaste Tree Berry experienced a significant decrease in the frequency and severity of hot flashes and other symptoms compared to those taking a placebo. Additionally, the herb's active compounds, such as agnuside and aucubin, are thought to contribute to its potential benefits.

Chaste Tree Berry is generally considered safe for most people, but it may cause side effects in some cases, including gastrointestinal upset, headaches, or skin reactions. As with any herbal supplement, it's important to consult with a healthcare provider before starting Chaste Tree Berry, particularly if you are taking other medications or have existing health conditions.

For those considering Chaste Tree Berry for managing perimenopause symptoms, a *common dosage is 400-500 mg daily of a standardized extract, which should include a high concentration of aucubin.* The herb is typically best absorbed when taken between meals.

6. St. John's Wort

St. John's Wort (Hypericum perforatum) is a flowering plant native to Europe, commonly used for its potential to alleviate depression. It may also offer benefits for managing mood swings and irritability that can occur during perimenopause. This herb contains active compounds like hyperforin and is available in various forms, including teas, tablets, liquid extracts, and topical applications.

For perimenopausal women, St. John's Wort might help alleviate certain symptoms such as mood swings and irritability. Some studies suggest that it may also reduce other perimenopausal symptoms like hot flashes when used alone or in combination with herbs like black cohosh.

While St. John's Wort is noted for its effectiveness in treating mild to moderate depression, it is important to use it with caution due to its potential interactions with various medications. This herb can affect how other drugs work, leading to possible side effects or reduced effectiveness of certain treatments. Always consult a healthcare provider before starting St. John's Wort, especially if you are on other medications.

When used orally and for short-term periods (up to 12 weeks), St. John's Wort is generally considered safe. However, it may cause side effects, including, agitation and anxiety, dizziness, digestive issues like diarrhea, constipation, and stomach discomfort and dry mouth.

Additional side effects can include:
- Fatigue and insomnia
- Headache

- Increased sensitivity to sunlight (photosensitivity)

There is limited information on the safety of topical use of St. John's Wort. It is advised to avoid using it without the supervision of a doctor. If you're considering St. John's Wort for managing perimenopausal symptoms, discuss it with your healthcare provider to ensure it's appropriate for your situation and to prevent any potential interactions with other medications.

While these herbs are commonly used and have historical significance in managing menopausal symptoms, their effectiveness can vary, and they are not universally beneficial for everyone. Herbal remedies can interact with prescription medications and may have side effects, so it's essential to consult with a healthcare provider before starting any new herbal treatment. Personalized medical advice ensures that the chosen remedy complements your overall health strategy and minimizes potential risks.

Conclusion

As we reach the end of this book, it's clear that perimenopause is far more than a mere chapter in a woman's life. It's a complex and deeply personal journey, one that encompasses physical, emotional, and social dimensions. Each chapter of this book has shed light on various aspects of perimenopause, from understanding its onset and symptoms to navigating the profound changes it brings.

In Chapter 1, we began by embracing the change, tackling the challenge of understanding perimenopause and breaking the silence surrounding it. We confronted societal taboos and encouraged open conversations, recognizing that acknowledging and discussing this transition is crucial to navigating it effectively.

Chapter 2 provided practical guidance on managing the physical changes associated with perimenopause. From hormonal fluctuations and irregular periods to hot flashes, night sweats, and weight management, we explored a range of strategies and interventions. We learned that while the physical manifestations of perimenopause can be daunting, there are numerous ways to address and manage these symptoms with both lifestyle adjustments and medical support.

The emotional rollercoaster was the focus of Chapter 3, where we delved into mood swings, anxiety, brain fog and depression. We highlighted the importance of self-care and stress management, emphasizing that maintaining emotional well-being is just as vital as addressing physical symptoms. This chapter reinforced that emotional fluctuations are a natural part of the transition, and finding healthy coping mechanisms is essential for navigating these changes with resilience.

The rest of the chapters underscored the significance of nurturing relationships during perimenopause. We explored how to communicate effectively with loved ones, maintain intimacy and sexuality, and build a robust support network. Understanding and supporting one another through this journey can greatly enhance both personal and relational well-being.

We focused on lifestyle changes that support optimal well-being. We discussed the importance of nutrition, exercise, sleep hygiene, and self-care rituals. Adopting a balanced lifestyle not only helps manage perimenopausal symptoms but also promotes overall health and vitality.

Finally, we emphasized the importance of seeking medical support when needed. We examined when to consult healthcare professionals, the role of hormone replacement therapy (HRT), and the potential benefits of complementary and alternative therapies. This chapter highlighted the need for a personalized approach to treatment, combining medical advice with natural remedies and lifestyle adjustments to create a comprehensive plan for managing perimenopause.

Throughout this book, you have interacted with personal stories that have illustrated the diverse experiences of women navigating perimenopause. These narratives need to be a reminder that while each journey is unique, the challenges and triumphs shared can offer support and encouragement.

As you move forward, remember that perimenopause is not an end but a new beginning. It's a time to embrace change, seek support, and prioritize your well-being. By integrating the knowledge and strategies shared in this book, you can approach this transition with confidence and grace. Ultimately, the journey through perimenopause is an opportunity for growth, self-discovery, and renewed strength. Embrace it with an open heart and a sense of empowerment, knowing that you have the tools and support to navigate this transformative phase with resilience and positivity.

References

Hawkins, A. L. (2012). *What you must know about Bioidentical hormone replacementtherapy: An alternative approach to effectively treating the symptoms of menopause.*

Hopsine, B. (2020). *Menopause: The causes, diagnosis, natural treatments and home solution for perimenopause, menopause, and Postmenopause.*

Menopause. (2022, October 17). World Health Organization (WHO). https://www.who.int/news-room/fact-sheets/detail/menopause

Perimenopause, early menopause symptoms | The North American Menopause Society, NAMS. (n.d.). North American Menopause Society (NAMS) - Focused on Providing Physicians, Practitioners & Women Menopause Information, Help & Treatment Insights.

https://www.menopause.org/for-women/menopauseflashes/menopause-symptoms-and-treatments/menopause-101-a-primer-for-the-perimenopausal

Perimenopause: Age, stages, signs, symptoms & treatment. (n.d.). Cleveland Clinic. https://my.clevelandclinic.org/health/diseases/21608-perimenopause

Perimenopause: Rocky road to menopause. (2022, August 9). Harvard Health. https://www.health.harvard.edu/womens-health/perimenopause-rocky-road-to-menopause

Samsioe, G. (1996). *Visual diagnosis self-tests on the menopause and HRT.*

Teaff, N. L., & Wiley, K. W. (1999). *Perimenopause: Preparing for the change : a guide to the early stages of menopause and beyond.* Harmony.

Whelan, N. (2005). *Perimenopause please: The psychological impact of perimenopause.* iUniverse.

Appendices

Appendix 1: Perimenopause Symptom Tracker

Tracking your symptoms during perimenopause can be incredibly useful for understanding how this transition is impacting you and for managing your health effectively. This symptom tracker will help you monitor changes, evaluate what strategies are working, and identify areas where adjustments might be needed in your treatment plan. It's a good idea to share this information with your healthcare provider during your appointments to guide discussions and decision-making.

How to Use the Tracker

1. Record your symptoms - Note down any symptoms you experience each day, including their intensity and duration.
2. Track your management strategies - Document the methods you're using to manage each symptom, such as lifestyle changes, medications, or other treatments.
3. Evaluate effectiveness - Regularly review which strategies are working and which might need adjustments.
4. Update your Plan - Based on your observations, make notes about potential changes to discuss with your healthcare provider.

Symptom Tracker Table

Date	Symptom	Severity (1-10)	Duration	Management Strategies	Effectiveness (1-10)	Notes/ Changes
Example:	Hot Flashes	7	30 minutes	Drunk cold water, wear light clothes	5	Consider discussing medication options
Example:	Mood Swings	6	Throughout the day	Practiced deep breathing exercises	7	Explore therapy options
Example:	Sleep Disturbances	8	1-2 hours	Avoided caffeine in the afternoon	6	Evaluate sleep hygiene techniques
Example:	Joint Pain	5	Occasional	Regular exercise, took anti-inflammatory supplements	4	Assess need for physical therapy

Tips for Effective Tracking

- Be Consistent - Record your symptoms daily to get an accurate picture of your perimenopausal experience.

- Be detailed - Include specifics about the severity, duration, and your management strategies for a comprehensive view.
- Review regularly - Regularly assess your entries to identify patterns and areas for improvement.
- Communicate with your healthcare provider - Bring your completed tracker to your appointments to facilitate productive discussions about your symptoms and treatment plan.

This symptom tracker is a valuable tool for managing your perimenopause journey, helping you to stay informed and proactive about your health.

Appendix 2: Questions for Your Healthcare Provider

When visiting your healthcare provider, having a list of questions can help ensure you get the information you need. Here are some important questions you might consider asking to guide your discussion about perimenopause: (Bringing these questions to your appointment can help you better understand your situation and explore the most appropriate treatment and management strategies.)

1. Do you regularly treat patients going through perimenopause, or should I see a specialist?
2. How can I distinguish between symptoms related to perimenopause and those caused by other health conditions?
3. What is the typical duration of perimenopausal symptoms, and how might menopause impact my overall health?
4. How long should I continue using birth control during perimenopause? Do I need any specific

treatments for menopause, and if so, what options are recommended for me?

5. Is hormone replacement therapy (HRT) a suitable option for me? What potential side effects should I be aware of, and how can I manage them?

6. How safe is hormone therapy for my health? What changes might I expect in my sexual health as I go through menopause?

7. How might menopause impact any existing health conditions or diseases I have?

8. Does menopause increase my risk for other health issues? What tests or screenings should I schedule, and how often should I have them?

9. Are there any specific medications, supplements, or natural remedies you suggest for managing perimenopausal symptoms?

10. Should I adjust my diet or exercise routine during perimenopause? What type and amount of physical activity are beneficial?

11. Are there any particular lifestyle changes that could be especially helpful during this transition?

12. How long does perimenopause generally last, and what signs will indicate that I have moved past it?

Appendix 3: Medication Tracker

Keeping track of your medications—whether they are prescription drugs, over-the-counter remedies, or dietary and herbal supplements—is crucial for managing your symptoms effectively. Use this medication tracker to monitor your regimen and ensure you're following your healthcare provider's instructions accurately. Place this tracker somewhere visible, like on your refrigerator or inside your medicine cabinet, to help you stay organized.

Medication Tracker

Medica-tion/Sup-plement	Dosage	Frequency	Time of Day	Instruc-tions	Notes/Side Effects
Example: Estradiol	1 mg	Daily	Morning	Take with food	None
Example: Calcium	500 mg	Twice daily	Morning & Evening	Take with water	Possible constipation
Example: Vitamin D	1000 IU	Daily	Evening	Take with meal	None
Example: Omega-3	1000 mg	Daily	With dinner	Take with food	Fishy aftertaste

How to Use This Tracker

- List all medications - Include all prescription and over-the-counter medications, as well as any dietary or herbal supplements you are taking.

- Enter dosage and frequency -Record the amount you need to take and how often.
- Specify time of day - Note the best time to take each medication, if applicable.
- Add instructions - Include any special instructions, such as taking with food or avoiding certain activities.

Monitor notes/side effects - Track any side effects or interactions you experience and any additional notes for your reference.

Important Tips

- Take your medications exactly as prescribed by your healthcare provider.
- If you experience any side effects or have concerns about interactions, discuss them with your healthcare provider before making any changes.

Only adjust or discontinue any medication with the guidance of your healthcare provider.

By keeping this tracker updated and sharing it with your healthcare team, you can ensure a more effective and safer management of your perimenopausal symptoms.

Appendix 4: Relaxation Techniques

Incorporating relaxation techniques into your routine can help alleviate both the physical and emotional strains of perimenopause. Here are some more effective methods to help you unwind and bring a sense of calm to your daily life:

Breathing Techniques

1. Rhythmic Breathing
   - Find a quiet place where you can sit comfortably.
   - Inhale slowly through your nose for a count of five, then exhale gently through your mouth for the same count.
   - Focus on the sensation of your breath entering and leaving your body, and how it affects your overall sense of relaxation.
2. Deep Breathing
   - Place your attention on your navel. Breathe in deeply, directing the air towards your abdomen.
   - Allow the breath to rise through your chest and shoulders. Exhale slowly as if you were deflating a balloon.
   - Repeat this process, observing how your body feels as you breathe in and out.
3. Visualized Breathing
   - Sit comfortably and close your eyes.
   - As you breathe in slowly, visualize a wave of relaxation flowing into your body. As you exhale, imagine stress and tension leaving your body.
   - Maintain a smooth, steady rhythm as you breathe deeply, visualizing relaxation filling you with each inhale and stress exiting with each exhale.
4. Progressive Muscle Relaxation
   - Focus on your breathing—inhale deeply and exhale slowly.

- Conduct a mental scan of your body, noting any areas of tension or tightness.
- Direct your breath towards these tense areas, visualizing the stress melting away with each exhale.
- Start at your toes and work your way up, allowing each muscle group to relax as you breathe deeply.

Additional Techniques

- Acupuncture and massage - Many women find relief from tension and stress through acupuncture and therapeutic massage. These practices can help soothe both body and mind.
- Yoga and Tai Chi - These gentle, mindful movements combine physical exercise with relaxation techniques, promoting overall well-being and reducing stress.